DR. SUZANNE STEINBAUM'S

HEART BOOK

AVERY

a member of

Penguin Group (USA) Inc.

New York

DR. SUZANNE STEINBAUM'S

HEART BOOK

Every Woman's Guide
to a Heart-Healthy Life

DR. SUZANNE STEINBAUM
with EVE ADAMSON

AVERY

Published by the Penguin Group
Penguin Group (USA) Inc., 375 Hudson Street, New York, New York 10014, USA • Penguin Group
(Canada), 90 Eglinton Avenue East, Suite 700, Toronto, Ontario M4P 2Y3, Canada (a division of
Pearson Penguin Canada Inc.) • Penguin Books Ltd, 80 Strand, London WC2R 0RL, England •
Penguin Ireland, 25 St Stephen's Green, Dublin 2, Ireland (a division of Penguin Books Ltd) •
Penguin Group (Australia), 707 Collins Street, Melbourne, Victoria 3008, Australia (a division of
Pearson Australia Group Pty Ltd) • Penguin Books India Pvt Ltd, 11 Community Centre,
Panchsheel Park, New Delhi–110 017, India • Penguin Group (NZ), 67 Apollo Drive, Rosedale,
Auckland 0632, New Zealand (a division of Pearson New Zealand Ltd) • Penguin Books (South Africa),
Rosebank Office Park, 181 Jan Smuts Avenue, Parktown North 2193, South Africa • Penguin China,
B7 Jiaming Center, 27 East Third Ring Road North, Chaoyang District, Beijing 100020, China

Penguin Books Ltd, Registered Offices: 80 Strand, London WC2R 0RL, England

Most Avery books are available at special quantity discounts for bulk purchase for sales promotions,
premiums, fund-raising, and educational needs. Special books or book excerpts also can be created to fit
specific needs. For details, write Penguin Group (USA) Inc. Special Markets, 375 Hudson Street, New York,
NY 10014.

Library of Congress Cataloging-in-Publication Data

Steinbaum, Suzanne.
Dr. Suzanne Steinbaum's heart book : every woman's guide to a heart-healthy life / Suzanne Steinbaum.
pages   cm
Includes index.
ISBN 978-1-58333-505-5
1. Heart diseases in women.   2. Women—Health and hygiene.   I. Title.   II. Title: Heart book.
RC682.S75   2013   2012039179
616.1'20082—dc23

Printed in the United States of America
1   3   5   7   9   10   8   6   4   2

Book design by Gretchen Achilles

Neither the publisher nor the authors are engaged in rendering professional advice or services to the
individual reader. The ideas, procedures, and suggestions contained in this book are not intended as a
substitute for consulting with your physician. All matters regarding your health require medical supervision.
Neither the authors nor the publisher shall be liable or responsible for any loss or damage allegedly arising
from any information or suggestion in this book.

While the authors have made every effort to provide accurate telephone numbers, Internet addresses, and
other contact information at the time of publication, neither the publisher nor the authors assume any
responsibility for errors, or for changes that occur after publication. Further, the publisher does not have
any control over and does not assume any responsibility for author or third-party websites or their content.

To Spencer Paul:
I learn from you and your beautiful heart every day.
I feel so lucky to be your mother—never forget that.
I love you from the bottom of my heart.

To Mom and Dad:
Never easy, but always worth it!
Without you, none of it could have happened.

To my patients:
Thank you for sharing your hearts with me.

Contents

PART TWO

WHAT YOU SHOULD DO

PART THREE

ALL ABOUT YOU

Acknowledgments

I would never be who I am without the influence and love of my grandparents: Pa and Ma and Grandma and Grandpa. I know you are smiling.

Dad: Everything you've ever taught me is right here in this book. Thank you for your time, effort, energy, and amazing edits at the perfect time. Mom: "Thank you" doesn't do it justice. There would have been no anything without you.

I have been so lucky to have "angels" step in and help make my dreams come true. Thank you, Annie Fox, my own special Tinkerbell, for teaching me *everything* and for always being there, no matter what, and Rusty Bergen for laying down the law and showing me the truth. To Ghylian Bell, my soul sister, whose path and mine were destined to cross, and Tony Leroy, who can make me laugh even when there is nothing to laugh about, who erased "victim" from the dictionary. For Brenda Strong, for being the light and my mirror, and for being that voice that every woman should be blessed to have.

My professional life would never be the same if it weren't for Dr. Steven Horowitz, my mentor and friend, and Dr. Gary Roubin, for having faith in me even when I was seven and a half months pregnant! And also my "lady doctor" girlfriends, without whom I might have just lost my way: Dr. Jill Kalman and Dr. Noelle Langan.

Finding a passionate crew like Pamela Serure and Carole Isenberg and the Events of the Heart made all the hard work have a place and a purpose, and of course I have to thank my American Heart Association family: Helaine Baruch, Amanda Loderstedt, Brooks Lancaster, Angie Harrison, and Megan Lozito. Thank you for making my world turn Red.

And to those whom I can never, ever thank enough: Jonnet and Peter Abeles, Alan Goldberg, Ron Shamask, Dr. Max Gomez, Cynthia Adler, Diane Terman, Renee and Al Chesley, and Virginia Hart. And to Martin Levine, sometimes cousin, sometimes doctor, and most always, a really good friend.

A special thanks to Pochea Ung. We will never have the words to describe what the passionate struggle has been like, and that the fort needed more than we could ever imagine. I will never stop reminding you how lucky we are.

A huge thank-you to Sarah Jane Freyman and Eve Adamson, who never turned away a morning report and another new story. To Peter Thall, who has been a cheerleader from the beginning.

A big thank-you to Megan Newman and Marisa Vigilante of Penguin Avery for really hearing me and believing that I could deliver the message.

A personal hug to Gary, Trang, Noah, and Matthew. To Jennifer, Jeremy, Max, and Simon, for being there for both of us, and playing with us! To Harvey, Stephannie, and Joshua, who are always there for us, no matter what.

Without Team Spencer, none of this book could have been written. With tons of love and appreciation for Daryl, Sarah, and Alexa Nanes. And, for always giving us a fabulous and fun place to play, Leslie Plaskon, JoAnn Difede, and Lucy Jo.

A special thought to Myra Weinstein, whose unconditional love will always be with me.

To my Aunt Phyllis, who put her heart in my hands from the beginning of my career and whose heart taught me not only about cardiology, but what personal strength and fortitude really mean.

A Dialogue with My
Five-Year-Old Son, Spencer

One morning, I was dictating some information for one of the chapters in this book, and my son, Spencer, grabbed the microphone from my hand and began to talk. He wanted to contribute his own thoughts to the book, and he was trying very hard to make it sound official. Now he calls it "our book," because he knows he is part of it. I hope you'll enjoy his wisdom.

SPENCER: I want Suzanne to take care of every people's heart.

SUZANNE: Why?

SPENCER: Because people need to take care of their own bodies and they have to eat good food and they will grow to be strong, healthy, and they exercise, by Suzanne Steinbaum.

SUZANNE: What's so important about exercise?

SPENCER: That you get healthy and you get exercise that you can lift double weight and you can do certain stuff that other people cannot do.

SUZANNE: And what does that do for your heart?

SPENCER: It keeps it healthy and your blood will be healthy and healthy, and you will be stronger than anything.

SUZANNE: That's great. Anything else you want to talk about when it comes to the heart?

SPENCER: My mom's book should be all sold out when she fixes everybody's heart.

SUZANNE: Thank you, Spencer. Anything else?

SPENCER: I have my mom take care of my dog and she has like a thousand people to take care of, so she has to do a lot of stuff to take care of everybody, like people in the medical hospital. The mommies have to take care of everybody so they're not sick. By Suzanne Steinbaum.

SUZANNE: Thank you, Spencer.

Introduction

We are heart-centered beings.

When I say that, I don't just mean that an organ we call the heart is located at approximately the center of our bodies, or even that our hearts are the engines that power our lives, although both of those statements are true. What I mean is something more. What I mean is the subject of this book.

We are also a head-centered culture. We live in our heads. Our thoughts race. We make checklists, and accomplish them. We are the CEOs of the lives we build, yet we have trouble calming down and being present. We are ambitious, active, and yes, exciting. We get things done, but we are also stressed out, burned out, and breaking down. Heart disease kills more women than all forms of cancer combined, and I believe, as a cardiologist, that the reasons for this go far beyond poor diet and lack of exercise (although those bad habits certainly contribute). I believe that the heartsickness I see in so many younger women today—the vague complaints, palpitations and panic attacks, the chest pains and fatigue and anxiety and sadness and general heaviness so many women feel—has everything to do with lives that have gone out of balance. We live in our heads. We are meant to live in our hearts.

Who a woman is, how she feels, what she projects to the world, what she takes inside her, her energy and love and compassion, all these things start inside and radiate out from the heart. This is true for some women more than others. Where one woman might feel stress or elation or anxiety in her stomach or back or head, many feel those most intense of human emotions in the heart. These women, I believe, are most vulnerable to heart disease later in life.

When you live in your head, you feel disconnected from your environment and your relationships, always talking, talking, talking to yourself. You get stressed, you don't sleep well, you may binge-eat or not eat at all. You gain weight in all the wrong places and before you know what hit you (because you aren't paying attention to your own needs), you are a miserable physical mess. When a doctor brushes you off by telling you that your symptoms are all in your head, in some ways, that doctor is right.

The problem is, your doctor may not tell you, when you are a young and vibrant thirty-something or forty-something-year-old woman, that your palpitations, chest pains, stiff neck, poor diet, embarrassing lack of exercise, or the unrelenting stress under which you continue to function are having any effect at all on your beautiful heart. A doctor won't always say "It's all in your head." He or she may say you are "probably just under stress," and tell you to lose weight or exercise more (although many won't even say that). Some may just tell you they don't know what's wrong with you at all. They might even make you feel like you are going crazy.

Even women in their fifties or sixties whose risk of heart disease goes up (we know for a fact it does) are often told by doctors that their vague symptoms are anything but their hearts. Maybe it's menopause, stress, anxiety, or the effects of life changes, like losing a spouse or retiring. But to you, it feels like something more.

I know what's wrong with you, and *it's not in your head. It's in your heart.*

I would never want you to accept such a "diagnosis," because even if your symptoms originate from a life lived out of the head, you deserve help and understanding in order to get yourself back into your center. That is why I wrote this book—to be a hand reaching out to help you. I see the first signs of heart disease in women decades before they ever have a heart attack, and your so-called vague complaints may just be your heart calling out for attention *now*, before it's too late. This is a book to help you get out of your head and find what's in your heart. Get out of your head and into your heart, and make yourself well.

Who I Am and Why I Believe You Can Heal Yourself

Eighteen people in my family are doctors. But we're not just doctors. We are doctors of osteopathic medicine, with the medical degree D.O. Doctors of osteopathy can prescribe medications, perform surgery, and use all the technology an M.D. can use, but the focus is very different—it is a very hands-on, personal way of doctoring that champions health promotion and disease prevention, rather than just treating symptoms or managing diseases.

This started with my grandfather, David Steinbaum. On a shelf in my office, I have the shingle my grandfather first hung outside his office in 1930, when he was 22, to remind me of my family's long tradition in preventative care. As a young boy living in Bayonne, New Jersey, David was told that he had a heart murmur, and that he was not allowed to play sports, specifically football. He was told he was sick. But my grandfather didn't feel sick, so he grew up suspicious of this notion that something was wrong with him. He believed he was fine. Not only that, but he grew up determined to find out more about his own body than that doctor could possibly tell him. So, after high school, he started taking courses on health and nutrition in New York City. Legend has it that a famous nutritionist encouraged my grandfather to look into osteopathy as his faith in traditional medicine waned.

So my grandfather studied and researched and learned all he could about osteopathic medicine. This was a minority profession at the time, with only five schools of osteopathy in existence (there are currently twenty-nine), so he opted to go to the founding school in Kirksville, Missouri. He went off to study osteopathic medicine, then came back to New Jersey to practice.

At that time, people didn't understand what kind of doctor he was, and they certainly didn't understand this curious "holistic approach" to medicine. He was passionate about teaching as well as about being a doctor, and he loved academics. In his spare time, he taught medically based basic science classes in a college in New York and took the national board exams required by M.D.s and D.O.s in order to practice in multiple states. Then he started writing articles.

When I began my medical training and became interested in preventive cardiology, my grandmother handed me some of my grandfather's old articles. I was stunned. Decades before any of this was in the news, my grandfather had written articles about the benefits of dark chocolate, blueberries, avocados, green leafy vegetables, and almonds on health. He'd written about antioxidants before that was ever a buzzword, and a passion for nutrition and healthy living long before it became fashionable. I read the articles again and again. "How is this possible?" I kept asking myself. I'd never talked to my grandfather about these subjects, but before all the research on the benefits of these foods, he knew. He'd known for sixty years. That was an important moment for me, to see myself as part of a lineage. I grew up in a family and in an environment where everyone assumed the body was meant to heal itself, and that each component, each part, fit together in a way that, if optimized, would promote proper function and healing. When the system broke down, when the body couldn't heal itself, then we were lucky to have medications and surgeries and all of those other things to deal with disease, but the first line of defense was optimizing the body's health by providing all the tools it needs to be as healthy as it can be. When I was deciding what kind of doctor I wanted to be, I realized I could not practice apart from this philosophy. It was too much a part of me. When you are raised with a certain belief system, whether it is a religion or a science or a way of living, it becomes ingrained in your psyche, and this is exactly how I felt about preventive care. My grandfather was so passionate about what he did that eighteen family members followed in his very big footsteps, and we all felt the same way: the body could heal itself. We just had to help people stop getting in the way of their own healing.

My grandfather believed in helping everyone he could, whether they could afford medicine or not. His door was always open. His office was connected to the house, and my playroom was in his office—patients seemed to love that I was there, even though I imagine I probably did get in the way sometimes. I had a book in which I wrote the names of my own pretend patients with their pretend diagnoses and their pretend treatments. I felt so official and important with my little book. Whenever I would go to my grandfather's house, I would run right into the office, ready to get to work. At three years old, I remember saying to my grandmother, "When am I going to learn how to read? I want to give eye exams." So my grandfather taught me the alphabet, not because I wanted to read books, but so I could help him give eye exams to his *real* patients. That was so exciting for me. I grew up with those patients. I knew them. They felt like part of the family, coming to the house, coming to my playroom for help.

At first, my father went into practice with my grandfather, and then he, on the strength of my grandfather's encouragement, came to

New York City and was accepted into a fellowship at Sloan Kettering, one of the most prestigious oncology institutes in the world. My father became an oncologist with that same belief system my grandfather had bestowed upon us all—that his job was to facilitate healing by optimizing health in the body, while also taking advantage of standard oncology treatment methods. Every morning during his rounds, he brought along a nurse, a social worker, a Reiki practitioner (an alternative therapist who manually manipulates a patient's energy flow), and a nutritionist. He provided group support not only for the patients but for their families too. He treated cancer holistically, as a family disease.

When I was a child and my dad was home on the weekends, he'd say, "I'm going to the hospital to make rounds." I'd say, "Me too. I'm coming too." He always let me. I learned all the patients' names, I knew all their diagnoses. With my vast preschool experience in my grandfather's office, I felt more than comfortable doing those rounds with my father at the hospital. I felt *qualified*. Many years later, even before I was a physician, I remember diagnosing my father's patients (unofficially, of course). I felt so involved with them, so interested in what they were going through. My father, like his father, didn't separate these patients from our lives. They were always, and still continue to be, part of our family. I feel that way about my own patients.

In my family, we all joke that we know our number—whether we were the third, fourth, seventh, or twelfth doctor in the family. I am number fourteen. Once a drug rep asked if he could sponsor our family reunion. A pharmaceutical company sponsoring a family reunion—something's twisted about that for sure!

I went on to become an osteopathic physician like my grandfather and my father, and came back to New York to do my training as an internist and then a cardiologist. I became board certified as a D.O., then as an M.D., after doing a residency at Beth Israel Medical Center in New York. First I did a D.O. internship and an M.D./D.O. residency, a fellowship in preventive cardiology, and then an M.D. fellowship in cardiology. Then I got board certified in cardiology, and I've been a preventive cardiologist ever since, but the way my mission evolved shaped me and the way I have chosen to broadcast my message. It all began with a young girl doctor on Rollerblades.

Block Island Syndrome

Back many years ago, when I was still in training, long before I'd decided to become a cardiologist, I had a summer job as an intern, assisting the one and only doctor on Block Island. Block Island is a picturesque little piece of land just off the coast of Rhode Island, and a favorite vacation spot. It has gorgeous beaches at the base of rocky bluffs, lighthouses, magnificent vistas, and a constant breeze that makes the waters absolutely perfect for sailing. Each day, quaint ferries drop off their loads of tourists from Rhode Island, Connecticut, and New York.

Block Island is all the things you think of when you picture the perfectly relaxing and secluded New England–style vacation, and I couldn't believe my good luck in getting this job. I was ready to experience gorgeous weather, beautiful scenery, and happy relaxed families as my occasional patients. A beach vacation combined with a job that would further my newly minted career? Perfect!

I expected the obvious issues like sunburns and scraped knees, fishing hooks stuck in fingers, and Lyme disease. But that wasn't exactly all that happened.

During that summer on Block Island I had a parade of seemingly healthy women in their thirties and forties come into that doctor's office, and they all seemed to be complaining of the same things: chest pain, palpitations, exhaustion, and other heart symptoms.

Heart symptoms?

The doctor and I performed the routine tests on each female patient who came into our clinic. We did the requisite EKGs, but in every case, the results were normal. What was up? Why would these seemingly healthy, often wealthy, tanned, toned, and vacationing women have any issues with their hearts?

Determined to figure this out, I obsessively talked to the patients and researched the topic. I couldn't let it go. It seemed so strange and unexpected. Why were these women in the prime of life spending their vacations in a doctor's office while their husbands and children were outside getting the sunburns, scraped knees, and bug bites I'd expected to see in the clinic? The only common denominator I could find was that all of these women had stressful lives. They were busy, overextended, playing multiple roles, usually with great success. But as soon as they went on vacation—when the normally frenetic pace of their lives came to a grinding halt and they were expected to "just relax"—they fell apart. All the dysfunction going on in their bodies was suddenly becoming apparent because they had stopped moving and thinking and obsessing and achieving long enough to notice. All those stress hormones that had been propelling them forward to get through their frenetic days had nowhere to go, so they began to flow in the bloodstream, where they were wreaking havoc, causing hearts to race, blood pressures to rise, and chest pain. I began to call it Block Island Syndrome.

I now recognize that I was sensing a new kind of heart disease in the first generation after Gloria Steinem shook up the role of women in society as we knew it. I could also see it in myself and my colleagues—at the time, almost 50 percent of medical students were women, and I saw us all juggling everything. I remember thinking, "This is just going to get worse." I remember cramming for exams, then getting horrible colds after exams were over. I remember my colleagues working insane hours, then trying to juggle husbands and children and social lives. We reaped the benefits of women's liberation, but someone forgot to give us the handbook on how our new lives were supposed to work. No one prepared us for what it really means to be everywhere and do everything and also take care of ourselves. We try to have it all, but sometimes things fall through the cracks—important things, like our health, like our hearts! (I'll talk more about this later.)

I moved on to other clinics, other training, but I continued to see the doctors in charge dismissing heart disease in women who were falling apart. I also began to see women with heart symptoms completely unlike the typical ones we often see in men. I heard patients talk about their stressful lives, and I started to see a pattern. Modern life itself was becoming a risk factor for heart disease.

I soon began to develop a theory: that this surge of heartsickness in women is directly related to the way we've become increasingly entrenched in our brains, at the expense of our hearts. I understood that I was seeing something real and extremely significant—a connection between the way a woman chooses to live her life and the health of her heart—but I wasn't yet sure how to articulate it. It wasn't until later in my career that I would fully embrace this phenomenon and that it would propel me into my life's work.

A few years later, I was doing a fellowship at Beth Israel Medical Center in New York City, and I was on call every fourth night for thirty-six-hour shifts. This was a particularly stressful time in my life. I was trying to be a doctor, but I was also trying to be a girly-girl who loved high heels and pretty dresses and makeup and going on dates with boys. It was difficult to juggle my life within the confines of this very masculine profession and my desire to keep in touch with my feminine side. I was dating while maintaining my crazy schedule. I was working in high heels (I still do), wearing lipstick and bangle bracelets, and living on jellybeans and tons of coffee to keep myself awake. At the same time, I was practicing serious medicine. I was sleep-deprived and malnourished, and my brain rarely stopped. I never relaxed, and it showed. I could see it in my own face, on my skin, in my energy level.

Then I went on a short vacation to, of all places, Block Island. And I started having chest pain and heart palpitations.

That's when I realized that I had Block Island Syndrome—I was a young, healthy woman in the prime of my life, and I was finally on vacation, but instead of relaxing, I was having heart symptoms. I was the one sitting in the doctor's office.

I did all the tests I knew I was supposed to do, and everything looked okay, just as it had for those other women I'd once been so obsessed with understanding.

Finding My Calling

A few years later, as a young doctor, I was working at Beth Israel when a woman in her mid- to late forties had a heart attack in the emergency room. She had been sitting there for a long time, waiting to be seen. She wasn't my patient, but I'll never forget her. She kept complaining of pain, and they thought she had gastroenteritis. The stomach flu. As she waited, they gave her medicine for her stomach. Nobody even considered that it might be her heart, until the monitor started beeping indicating an irregular heart rhythm, and then she had a heart attack.

This woman was much too young to be having a heart attack, according to conventional medical "wisdom." Of course, nobody saw it coming, because why would they? We were all trained by the same system, and women her age simply didn't have heart attacks. She was an anomaly.

Or was she?

I never found out what happened to her, but I couldn't forget her because I watched the medical system fail her. We didn't help her because we didn't diagnose her in time. Maybe she recovered and maybe she didn't, but I already know that if she survived, she probably didn't get the same level of treatment and care she would have gotten if she were a man. The medical profession doesn't know as much about heart disease in women as they do about heart disease in men, and they knew even less back then than they do now. The research just wasn't there. I wanted to change all that. I wanted to change the perception of heart disease, and focus on preventing it in the first place. This became my passion. I believed that if people were given the lifestyle tools or proper medication, they would never get heart disease. This made heart disease different from cancer or kidney disease. I didn't want to help people who were sick, I wanted to help people stay healthy, and if they did get sick, then I wanted to help them reclaim that health. Quite frankly, I couldn't dream of a better profession. I decided I wanted to be a cardiologist, but one who could prevent heart disease rather than simply treat it.

I was lucky, because the chief of cardiology at Beth Israel, Dr. Steve Horowitz, had an interest in the effects of lifestyle on heart disease. He had collaborated with Dr. Dean Ornish and continued his work from Dr. Ornish's famous Lifestyle Heart Trial. The Beth Israel Center for Cardiac and Pulmonary Health offered a program of diet, exercise, group support, and stress management in the form of yoga, based on Dr. Ornish's trials. This was lifestyle intervention, for patients who already had evidence of heart disease. This aspect of prevention, from the place of behavioral changes and lifestyle choices, fascinated me.

I saw amazing things in that program. Maintaining a low-fat diet, exercising and doing yoga, and participating in group support, patients who already had heart disease were thriving. I got to observe firsthand the powerful effects of lifestyle changes on heart health. I watched people connecting with other people, and saw the difference this human connection made on heart function. I saw what it looked like when hearts mended themselves. This was also around the time that we began to understand that heart disease starts long before symptoms appear, and that it starts with damage to the lining of the arteries. This lining is called the endothelium, and I'll be mentioning it a lot in this book because it's so important that you understand what it is. The endothelium is the lining of your arteries, and its purpose is to protect your inner arterial wall. However, poor lifestyle choices like smoking and an unhealthy diet can damage the endothelium. Dr. Horowitz and I used to sit down together and brainstorm ways in which the endothelium could be protected, and how to manage people's behavior and choices so they wouldn't keep doing things that were eventually going to lead to heart disease. Through the Center for Cardiac Health, we saw people getting better, hearts getting stronger, cholesterol levels and blood pressures dropping, and weight decreasing. We knew that we were seeing the future, but we didn't know exactly when the science was going to catch up. At that point, exercise, diet, and stress reduction were still considered "alternative" medicine.

When my mentor and chief moved on, I took over his role as medical director of the Center for Cardiac Health. Those days were transformative, as Charles Leighton, the social worker who headed group support, taught me the power of communication for heart patients. I learned to read what patients with heart disease were feeling when their hearts got sick or failed them. I got more intuitive. I learned even more about the power of yoga and breathing, and especially exercise. I witnessed its transformative power over and over again. It led me to believe what I still repeat to my patients almost every day: "Exercise is the best medication."

But I still had more heart lessons to learn.

Facing My Own Heart

Fast-forward a few more years, when I came to Lenox Hill Hospital to run the Women and Heart Disease program. I started the job when I was seven and a half months pregnant. I was working at the hospital every night until 8:00, and even after I had my son (three weeks early, after just getting off work), I kept my insane schedule. I was doing it all—I was a busy cardiologist with a young son. But I was also losing it all.

I don't like to talk about this very often, but it's important for what happened next: My marriage was disintegrating and I didn't know how I was going to hold my life together. My stress level was unreal, but I kept pushing through, pretending I could handle it. I bet you know the feeling. I felt that I had no other choice but to keep going. It was almost as if I'd forgotten everything I'd learned about the importance of lifestyle and heart health. Somehow all that was theoretical, or applied only to my patients, not to me.

I remember being in the middle of a board meeting for Events of the Heart, a nonprofit organization committed to educating women about heart health through the creative arts. It was February, so it was during American Heart Month, and we were discussing the issues surrounding women and heart disease, when my heart started to race. I couldn't catch my breath, and it felt like my heart was coming out of my throat.

Being a cardiologist, I knew exactly what I was experiencing: supraventricular tachycardia. This is a condition in which the top part of your heart starts going too fast and the bottom part can't catch up. Of course, I knew what to do. I'm a cardiologist, after all. I did the proper maneuvers to make it stop, which include coughing, massaging my carotid artery, and even bearing down (like what you would do if you were pooping—trust me, it works). I did what I was supposed to, and eventually wore a monitor, and properly diagnosed myself. I experienced the problem intermittently for months. As long as my stress and heartsickness were at the forefront of my life, so was this new and disturbing heart condition.

Don't panic—not all palpitations signal a dangerous condition, and I'll talk much more about this later. However, I had to face the facts. Hearts aren't supposed to experience this. It's a sign that something is wrong. My heart was trying to get my attention, to shake me into alertness, forcing me to pay attention and get out of my head.

This was a huge wake-up call for me. I knew what was happening to my heart, but most women are not cardiologists, and I realized directly, in a way I never had before, exactly how it feels. If this happens to you (and it happens to many women), you might get scared, or panic, or you might ignore it. Even if you are diligent and see a doctor, that doctor might tell you it's nothing. That it's "just stress." Or that it's "all in your head."

When you are under great stress, whether from work or lost love or for any other reason, it can harm your heart as much as a poor diet or lack of exercise. I was brokenhearted in more ways than one, and that's when I realized exactly what it feels like. I realized, on a personal level, how emotions can affect the heart, and I knew that if it could happen to me, it could happen to anyone. I've lived with and worked with this knowledge ever since, spreading the word that heart disease *can happen to you,* and it likely will, unless you do something about it now.

The passion that I got from my father and from my grandfather remains very much in my heart and in my system. I want to help people understand what I've been learning since I was a child. I want to help people realize that there are things they can do to take care of their health, to keep themselves from developing the chronic diseases that have forced so many people to become dependent on medications and surgeries. I've seen it. I've seen generations of doctors, over decades of my own life, teaching patients how to take care of themselves. So I write this book in my own voice, but also with the voice of my grandfather, my father, and my whole family—all eighteen doctors, and the rest of the family, too, who have all lived with and grown to trust a system that says *you do not have to get sick.*

I tell this story because I want readers to understand what my perspective has been. It isn't new. It isn't something I came to when holistic health became a fad. It is in my blood, and in my system, and in my thought process. I have spent a lifetime witnessing healing from the inside out as a direct result of preventive and holistic care.

But the way I have put my own personal stamp on this mission is to apply it to your heart, because of all the organs in your body, I believe your heart is the center of it all, and when you live from it and for it, you will be in balance, and your body will know exactly what to do.

This is my mission, and I feel compelled to shout it from the rooftops, but the closest I can get to that is to write it in this book: Heart disease is about *you.* And *you* can do something about it. This book will show you how.

This book is divided into three parts. In the first part, "What You Should Know," I'll tell you what you should know about your heart, including your individual risk factors (I call these Heart Throbs) for heart disease, how your heart actually works, and how the medical establishment is likely to treat you if you should ever have any heart issues (or any health issues at all). In the second part, "What You Should Do," I'll give you the tools to start making changes in your own life, including how to start your own personal Heart Book, what medical tests you must know about, the best way to eat and exercise to prevent or reverse heart disease, and how to manage your own physical and psychosocial Heart Throbs. In the last part, "All About You," we'll get even more specific. I'll help you determine why you might have trouble sticking to your health plan, how to practice deep self-care, why your hormones may be messing with your mind, body, and heart, and how to handle the stress and anxiety that can come from personal tragedy.

This is a journey. I often say to my patients, "Welcome to boot camp!" because they have already developed heart disease. They've had their wake-up call. But I'd like you to join us in boot camp, *before* you get your wake-up call. This book is about changing your life, because I want you to be stronger, healthier, fitter, and more heart-led than you were before you took this journey with me. So get ready. Open your heart. This is what you need to know. This book could save your life. Do it for your family. Do it for yourself.

When you live in a way that is good for your heart, that comes from the heart, that puts the heart in charge, you'll live healthier, happier, fitter, and *longer*. You'll be more *you* in every fantastic way. Don't waste even one more heartbeat living in opposition to your most important body part. You're my patient now. Let's get you back to your best self.

PART ONE

What You Should Know

CHAPTER ONE

It's Not in Your Head—
It's in Your Heart

*But Mommy, why can't people
take care of their own hearts?*
—*my son,* SPENCER, *age 4*

This is a book about the heart, but more specifically, it is a book about *your* heart. Where is your heart? Do you lead with it, or hide it? Do you open it, or keep it shut? Do you live from it, or are you (as most of us are these days) typically stuck living from your head?

This isn't a book about heart disease. It isn't a medical book, although it contains medical information, and I do talk about heart disease. This is a *heart book*, and to me, that means much more than a "medical book."

I have a very specific reason for writing a heart book as opposed to a medical book. This is a book meant to *prevent* heart disease. It is a book for women who aren't yet diagnosed with heart disease. It is a book for women who may be at risk but don't know it, or who know it but don't want to think about it, or who believe they are too young to worry about it, or who think their healthy habits preclude it. It is a book for *you*. I want you to know more than you know right now about your heart, so you can take care of it better than you are taking care of it now. This is a book about changing your fate, and changing your life.

Over the years, I've often wished I could share patient stories so all women could benefit, and I've included some of these stories in this book, but they just keep coming. In fact, as I was finishing this book and thinking this first chapter was finished, I had two separate patients come into my office who perfectly exemplified the very *heart* of why I wrote this book, and I found I had to stop the presses and add their stories right here at the beginning, for your sake.

The first patient who came to see me is a 62-year-old woman. While she was in a rehabilitation center after having knee replacement surgery and receiving physical therapy, she began to get back pain. She complained to the doctors at the rehab center, and they told her it was muscular. After all, she'd just had surgery and she wasn't used to this level of exercise. They gave her a muscle relaxant, but the pain kept getting worse. Soon the pain was radiating down both sides of her back and down one shoulder and into her arm.

The pain was severe. She called her doctor while still in the hospital, and he told her it was indeed likely a muscular problem. Yet the pain kept increasing. Soon the pain was so bad that she called the nurse, crying hysterically, but the nurse simply assumed she was overreacting and refused to call the doctor again. It was decided. She was in the rehab center and it was clearly muscular. And now she was also considered a little crazy.

Finally, in despair, the woman called her husband, who drove to the hospital and demanded that the rehab center call an ambulance. This ambulance then drove her to the emergency room *in another hospital,* where this poor woman experienced sudden cardiac death, was resuscitated, and was then determined to have had a major heart attack.

This woman was healthy and active and was doing well after her knee surgery, so an important question is: Why did she have that heart attack? But just as important, I believe it is crucial to ask the question: *Why didn't anybody at that hospital help her?* This woman has two brothers who had heart bypass surgery in their forties and a sister who died of a stroke, but she looked healthy, so she seemed an unlikely candidate for heart disease. When I asked her, as I always ask my patients, "In your gut, deep down, did you know it was your heart?" she told me, "I had a feeling it was my heart, but I was afraid to say it out loud."

The other patient who came to see me recently is 37 years old and is an assistant director for a television show. Three months earlier, while she was working on the set, she almost passed out. She started sweating and had intense chest and arm pain. Her colleagues brought her to her trailer and urged her to go to the hospital, but she refused. She was busy! Her pain lasted for several hours, and then she went back to work.

The next day, she went to see her doctor, who didn't consider her symptoms an emergency but did recommend that she come see me. She did come to see me—*three months later.* Because she was busy. It was on her to-do list, but not only was she working fourteen-hour days, she was also driving three hours every weekend to see her mother, who needed to be taken up to Boston for cancer treatment. In addition, she was helping her single-parent sister raise a teenage son. She simply hadn't had time to make an appointment with me.

I did an echocardiogram on this woman and saw that her heart was working at a fraction of its full capacity. All evidence pointed to the fact that she had suffered a massive injury to her heart, and had not received any treatment for it. She was lucky to be alive. I ordered an invasive angiogram and a cardiac MRI to be sure before I broke the news to her. All she said was, "Should I be worried?"

What do you think? Of course she should be worried. She is under crushing stress. I asked if she had people to talk to, and she told me this: "I'm good at compartmentalizing." What I saw was a woman who had compartmentalized herself right into major heart disease. Her heart may never recover.

Either one of these women *could have been you.* Neither knew she had heart disease. Neither had prior symptoms. Neither was being evaluated for any heart issues. These women were both active, successful, healthy professionals who were not typical heart disease risks but who were living lives that predisposed them, without knowing it.

This is why I wrote this book. We need to do something about this problem. We all need to understand that these women's stories *are not unusual.* This is tragic, and preventable, and it must end. No woman should ever have to fight to get care for her heart; no woman should be afraid to speak up when she knows, with her intuition, that her heart is sick; and no woman should ever feel like she is too busy to take care of herself. Every woman should have enough understanding of her own heart, and of who she is, and of what she needs to be healthy and nurture her heart.

These are extreme examples of heartsickness, and yet they aren't all that extreme because heart disease exists on a spectrum and *most women today are headed in that same direction.* What I call "heartsickness" is rampant, and epidemic, and *curable,* and there are few things in my life more important than making sure every woman understands this message and knows how to go in a different direction, so heart disease won't keep happening. I don't ever want heart disease to happen to you. I want you to live a strong, healthy, vital life well into old age.

But chances are, heart disease will be a part of your life. As a preventive cardiologist, I see women in my New York City office every day who are heartsick. They may suffer from minor complaints or major ones, but overall, the pattern I see emerging, the pattern that alarms me and my colleagues, is an increasing rate of heart disease and disability in women at younger and younger ages. Heart disease is the disease most likely to kill you, and yet, as doctors, sometimes we miss it, because heart disease doesn't always look the same in women as it does in men, or because we simply don't expect to see it in someone as young as, say, 37. Or even 60.

It doesn't matter how old you are. We know that statistically, women in their fifties, sixties, and seventies are more prone to heart attacks than women in their twenties, thirties, and forties. We know, in general, that heart disease develops about ten years after menopause, and about ten years later than it does in men, but that's in the general population. Those are statistics, but *you are not a statistic*. I'll say this again and again.

What matters to me, and what should matter to you, is you and your heart. What I want you to learn from this book, more than anything else, is that heart disease is not somebody else's problem. It *can* happen to you, even if you don't have the classic risk factors, even if you don't have a family history, even if you don't believe it.

This book pertains to women at risk for heart disease, but it also pertains, equally so, to those who don't think they are at risk. It is for women in their fifties and sixties and seventies, but it is also for women in their twenties and thirties and forties. It is for us all. We are all at risk. Modern life puts us at risk. Modern diets put us at risk. Modern conveniences put us at risk. Just existing in this society as it is puts us at risk.

I believe I have a relatively unique perspective on heart disease in women, because as a preventive cardiologist, part of my job is to see heart disease happening before it is clinically present and before any indication of heart disease will show up on any test. I see it every day, and this is what I see: distraction, stress, sleeplessness, anxiety, and depression. I see people living lives that aren't the lives they really want to live. I see people who can't find their passions, or who can't find equilibrium in their relationships, who suffer because of tragedies from the past, or who can't seem to find the will to establish healthy habits. I see people who barely recognize themselves in the mirror anymore. I see imbalance.

I believe this imbalance comes from a lack of heart-centeredness. Our hearts know exactly what we want and need. Why have we sidelined them? Why do we diminish their importance? And how can we turn that harmful habit around?

By getting out of our heads, and learning how to live from our hearts.

Living from the Heart

Living from the heart feels much different from living from the head. When you live from your heart, you feel at peace, at ease, and in control of yourself because of a deep inner knowing. You lead with love. You learn how to care for yourself and love yourself. You relax because you know that everything is going to be okay. Living from the heart coaxes your body back into balance. When the heart is in control, your body finds optimum health and starts acting like a well-oiled machine instead of a broken-down car.

We are so used to letting our heads be in charge of our lives that when we start reacting with our hearts instead, it feels like a miracle, like a whole new existence. And it is! The heart is the center of our body's universe and the center of our feelings. This is as it should be. Your head is way off at the edge of your body. You can't balance when you are living from there. Your head isn't grounded in the reality of your body. Let your heart be the center and watch your whole life transform.

This is a book about how to do exactly that—how to get out of your head and live from your heart by learning to care for and nurture your most crucial and central of internal organs. This is your handbook and your guide for creating a heart-centered life. It's about heart health, but it's also about so much more. It's about your *life*, and every aspect of your life that can and will influence your heart, for better or for worse.

You store everything you love inside that heart, and you also store things you don't love. You've got a lot going on in there, and that's why nurturing your heart is so crucial. If you aren't paying attention, you will get sick one day. By learning to put your heart first, you can actually stop the disease process now, when it's still easy to do. What's more, you'll get in better shape. You'll have more energy. You'll look better. You'll lose weight. You'll feel calmer and more in control of your life.

I am writing this book because this is the book I want to read. This is the voice of your future, looking back and saying, "Be careful what you do." This is the voice saying, "I've seen what's coming for you, and you want to take a different road. You're on a collision course. Take this exit."

Your heart is always trying to tell you something about your bigger picture. It will lead you in the right direction in your life. Your heart is wise. Are you listening?

Hundreds of thousands of people like you will die from heart disease this year, and next year, and the year after that. It's happening. It's epidemic. But it has a cure. I want to tell *you* how to stop it, because you, better than anyone else, better than any doctor, can affect your own chances for developing heart disease and dying from a heart attack. You can take your heart into your own hands and stop the disease process in your own body, the one that has likely already begun.

Because if you are overweight, you have heart disease. If you don't eat very well, you have heart disease. If you don't exercise on most days, if you are depressed, if you don't get enough sleep, you have heart disease. If you have high blood pressure or high cholesterol, if you bum cigarettes off friends or eat too much or don't sleep enough or suffer from anxiety or never exercise, you are already heartsick. It is just a matter of time before you know it. Before it shows.

You are barreling straight toward a serious future illness, and your body is already logging the damage. You are flirting with heart disease. You are courting heart disease. Heart disease is already on your radar. I want to change that outcome. I want to help you turn things around, before it's too late. I want to tell you this *now*, before you get sick, and maybe it will help motivate you to do something.

I think heart disease needs to be redefined by all of these issues in your life. You may not have heart disease according to the standard definition as established by the medical community, but heart disease starts long before it manifests as pathological. Your heart, and by extension your entire life, can be better than it is today. Even if it can't yet be measured through a blood test, you are on a slippery slope, my friend. It's time to climb back up to a place of strength, energy, radiance, beauty, and health. It's time to become fully and proudly heart-centered.

Just by picking up this book, you are taking the first step, tapping into the wisdom of your heart to know yourself better. You are changing your outcome. Just by accepting the potential of disaster and proactively doing something about it, you are increasing your odds of future heart health, longevity, and most important, vitality. The voice in this book constantly reminds you what it means to stay on *your* course, your path. It reminds you that it's *your* heart, and you know best when it's not doing well, and when it's thriving. It encourages you to live fully, with health and vitality, from the center of your universe. It encourages you to live from your heart.

And you will be vastly less inclined to have a heart attack. Ever. You can stop that slow progression toward heart disease that may already be in progress. You might just be able to foil the number-one killer in both women and men.

Knowing Your Heart

Women are naturally heart-centered beings, with intuitions and sensitive systems that speak to them, if only they will listen. When I look at a woman who has come into my office because of palpitations or chest pain, or even because of anxiety or exhaustion, I listen to her heart, but I don't just listen to the physical heart. I listen to what she has to say, and how she says it—I listen to her emotional heart. I look for vitality. I look for balance. I look for calm, for joy, for the signs of a deep inner wellness.

I also look for signs that the heart has to work harder than normal to do something simple, like climb a flight of stairs or walk around the block. I ask about how she sleeps, how she likes her job, how content she is in her relationships. I ask about what she feeds herself, how much she moves her body, how much support she has, what she loves. I ask about her passions. I ask about her heart in the bigger sense of that word, beyond the physical internal organ pumping blood and oxygen through her body.

You can do this for yourself. You can ask these questions for yourself. Do you feel vital, balanced, calm, joyful? Can you climb the stairs, walk around the block? How do you sleep? How are your relationships? What do you eat? How much do you move? What do you love? What are your passions? This book will guide you.

Of course, you should also get the medical care you need. I would never dismiss or discount what modern medicine does. Cardiology research has taught us so much we didn't know before that we are now able to catch and treat hundreds of thousands of cases of heart disease in men and women, and we are able to save lives in ways we couldn't even dream of decades before. But there is still so much we don't know, especially when it comes to women's hearts. We are moving in the right direction, sometimes, but still there are great gaps in our knowledge, and the learning curve is shallow. Answers aren't coming fast enough for me, and I'm not patient!

There is a reason for this, and it has to do with the way our medical system is set up. I'll talk about this in more detail later, but the simple fact is that modern medicine is about public health. This is by necessity. Research scientists need to look at the numbers, and the risk-benefit analysis, and what will help most of the people most of the time—as far as they can estimate. It's the most practical way to help a large population, and it is effective, in many cases.

But that's not what health means to *you*. You aren't a statistic. Your treatment plan doesn't necessarily need to be based on a risk-benefit analysis. To you, health is about your real life, what you are able to do every day, how you feel, and what you can give to others. It's about your physical and emotional and metaphorical heart. Is it going to be there for you when you need it most? Or is it going to fail you? You don't necessarily want to know what's going to happen to *most people*. You want to know what's going to happen to *you*, and what *you* can do about it.

Here's the fact: Heart disease is the number-one killer of women. Here are more facts:

- A woman dies about once every minute in the United States from cardiovascular disease.

- More women die from heart disease than all forms of cancer, chronic lower respiratory disease, Alzheimer's disease, and accidents combined.

- Recently, heart disease rates have started to rise for women ages 35 to 54—an age when most women aren't even thinking about heart disease yet.

- By the age of 60, half of us will have heart disease.

- A third of African American women suffer from hypertension even before they hit 60.

- Forty-five percent of our population has high blood pressure, high cholesterol, or diabetes—all major risk factors for heart disease.

- Heart disease rates in men under 55 are falling, but in women under 55, they are rising.

- In those women who do have heart disease, the disease process didn't start on the day of the heart attack. It started years, *decades* before.

These are public health statistics, but they are also statistics about you, because no matter how strong and well you guess your heart is right now, this is the disease most likely to end your life, or sap your vitality so that your future years will be more about disability and pain than joy and contentment.

The good news is, despite how much we don't know, despite how much any individual's heart symptoms may be overlooked, despite the daunting numbers, for you, right here, right now, and for your heart, beating right there in the center of your chest, there is a solution.

Your doctor doesn't have all the answers. Your doctor might not tell you what's coming, and probably won't, because your doctor doesn't know. He can quote statistics for you, but he can't predict your individual future. And when heart dysfunction does come, he might not catch it in time. He might not see how heart disease will manifest in *you*. (I tend to use "he" when I refer to doctors, just because it's simpler, so please don't assume I am being sexist or making any favorable or unfavorable assumptions about male doctors. They are the people in my family, remember?)

This goes against everything we've been taught to believe. People think the doctor is the ultimate authority, and we doctors do know a lot about certain things—things we trained for, things you likely don't know. But when it comes to the nature of your own heart, *you* are the answer to the problem of heartsickness because *you can heal your own heart,* and no one else can possibly know your heart better than you. Your doctor can help, of course, with tests and diagnoses and advice, but only you can change direction. You can change your world. Eighty to 90 percent of the time, heart disease is preventable, but preventing it is up to you. This book will show you how.

Heart disease is the destiny of most Americans, and yes, there is a standard of care for heart patients. Yes, there are known risk factors for heart disease, and those are very important. They are your first line of defense. There are proven lifestyle changes you can make to reduce your risk of heart disease, and they are very important too. There are things you should know if you are postmenopausal and at an increased risk for heart disease, and this is crucial.

But I'm talking about more than the standard of care, the known risk factors, and the proven lifestyle changes. I'm talking to all women, of every age—and men, too. And I'm talking about your *life,* how you choose to live it, how you choose to view the world, how you choose to conduct your relationships, how you choose to see yourself in the mirror, what you choose to do and who you choose to be. I'm going to talk about your heart, not just literally but metaphorically. I'm going to show you exactly why you need to be concerned about it, and why you—at any age—can make changes now that will make all the difference in the world later. I'm going to ask you to think about your heart. What role does it play in your life? And then I'm going to ask you to make some changes.

Your Heart

I see women of all ages in my office, but the symptoms or conditions I'm seeing with increasing frequency in premenopausal women who aren't typically being screened for heart disease yet include:

- Chest pain
- Shortness of breath
- Heart palpitations
- Dizziness, lightheadedness, or fainting
- Exhaustion or fatigue
- Anxiety
- High blood pressure
- High cholesterol
- High triglycerides
- Elevated hemoglobin A1C
- Plaque in the arteries
- Obesity
- Metabolic syndrome (a precursor to diabetes)

Why Doctors Aren't Helping You

Now let's talk about another aspect of this problem. Let's talk about that first woman I told you about at the beginning of the chapter, the one who was in a hospital having a heart attack and couldn't get anyone to treat her. Why is this happening? Why are women's heart problems seemingly marginalized? If you don't understand the big picture about this issue, you won't be in the best position to get the help you need, so I want you to have some important information on this subject.

When I am giving talks in my role as a national spokesperson for Go Red For Women of the American Heart Association, I often get asked questions like, "Why are doctors deliberately ignoring this issue?" and "Why aren't there studies about women's hearts?" and "Why don't they care about us?" These questions imply that we, as women, are the victims, but let me at least reassure you that we aren't victims. There is no vast cardiology conspiracy against women. We are simply the by-products of a medical system that is trying to catch up with reality. There are many reasons why this is the case. Women were an afterthought in cardiac research for a long time, not because they were trying to ignore us, but because the medical establishment actually believed that heart disease was a male problem and that women didn't usually suffer from it. At the very first American Heart Association conference in 1965, there was a session for women entitled "How to Take Care of Your Man's Heart." Isn't that amazing?

But it wasn't a conscious omission, just lack of knowledge. It wasn't until 1994, when the Office of Women's Health in Washington, D.C., was established as part of the U.S. Food and Drug Administration, that the government required 50 percent of the populations in any government-funded study to be women. When you write a grant now, you have to include a separate piece of paper that states that every effort will be made to include women and minorities in your study. It is only recently that this change has affected the standard of care, because it takes a long time to conduct research, evaluate it, and integrate it into the health-care system. It can take twenty years to change the way we look at things and integrate that change into the standard of care. And those are only the studies funded by the government. In cardiology journals that publish studies funded privately or by industry, women are included in the research for those studies only about 23 percent of the time, and in internal medicine journals, women are included in studies only about 37 percent of the time. But again, there are reasons for this. Many women do not participate in trials because they are too busy, unable to commit, don't see the value, or put themselves last. We often don't have the women we need in order to conduct a legitimate trial! Also, because women can get pregnant, they are often necessarily excluded, for safety reasons. Or gender is simply not the important demographic in the study. Everyone is lumped together.

Another important thing to consider is that women's lives have changed, so our hearts have changed too. Heart disease actually *is* more of a problem for women than it used to be, probably because we are living lives that are more like men's lives now, with the heavy pressures of earning a living but with the added pressures of also taking care of families. We are having more heart disease than before, so it really is more of a problem than it was (although heart disease has *always* afflicted women). Women move at the speed of light, and modern medicine sometimes seems to move at the speed of molasses, so it's no wonder we've left science behind.

In the meantime, as science is catching up, when a woman does have heart disease, the data from the trials and studies that were mostly about men are what doctors use, and then they have to extrapolate the results to women in order to treat them. However, since women's hearts don't always behave like men's hearts, those extrapolations aren't always going to be correct. In many cases, they may be dead wrong. We have no choice but to treat women with the data we have available right now, and unfortunately, that means we aren't always going to do a very good job.

Because of the lack of information, the viewpoints of doctors and patients, the difficulty in diagnosing, and the subtle symptoms, fewer women than men are referred to tests for the heart, such as angiograms, and fewer women are given lifesaving procedures such as by-pass surgery or stenting, or are referred for implantable defibrillators. Even fewer are given the lifesaving medications we use after heart disease such as atherosclerosis has been diagnosed. We simply don't have the data on women. And that means we may not know how to treat them, let alone diagnose them. Forget the fact that I'm a doctor—I'm also a woman, and as a woman, this reality is a little scary to me too!

On top of all that, most women aren't even being treated by cardiologists. Although even the most well-trained cardiologists in the country still don't have all the answers, it's important to recognize that for most women, their primary care doctor is more likely to be their ob-gyn or internist. Unfortunately, only 40 to 50 percent of these doctors are aware of the cardiovascular disease prevention guidelines formulated just for women, which weren't even established until 2002 and which were revised to reflect continuing research in 2007 and again in 2011. In the scheme of medicine, this is like yesterday. More internists might have an understanding of the risk of heart disease for women, but still, only a relatively small percentage of them actually recommend prevention practices for their patients. Because of this, heart disease in women is misdiagnosed, not as aggressively treated, and not as equally prevented as it is in men.

Women themselves know even less. Not only do the doctors not know how to diagnose and treat heart disease in women, but the patients are equally unaware. Based on national statistics, only 66 percent of white women know that heart disease is their number-one health threat. Only 43 percent of African American women and 44 percent of Hispanic women know this information. So, you see, we are in trouble on both ends.

There is another problem—not only do women not know that heart disease is an issue for them, but they are actually dying from coronary artery disease without ever knowing they have it. In one study, the first symptom of heart disease was sudden cardiac death in 64 percent of women and 50 percent of men. And when women do get heart disease and live with it, they don't do as well. In this same study, one year after having a heart attack, 25 percent of men died, whereas 38 percent of women died.

Sudden cardiac death. I don't want to alarm you, but . . .

Actually, I *do* want to alarm you. Because if we are not alarmed, what will make us change? What will make us take our futures into our own hands?

WomenHeart: The National Coalition for Women with Heart Disease and the Society for Women's Health Research recently released a report that lists the top ten questions we still have regarding the cardiovascular care of women—important questions *we still haven't answered.* I'm going to address these throughout this book, but I'd like you to start thinking about them now. I've reworded them in layperson's terms to make them more accessible:

1. Why does heart disease develop differently in women than in men, and why do women fare more poorly than men when they have heart disease?

2. What can we do to prevent heart disease in women, or to diagnose it early?

3. How can we better assess symptoms of heart disease in women, especially those symptoms that are less typical, since women often don't have the most obvious symptoms, such as chest pain?

4. What role do hormones play in the development of heart disease in women, specifically as may relate to menstrual history, pregnancy history, and hormone replacement therapy?

5. What specific issues of pregnancy increase the risk of cardio-vascular disease, and how can we best diagnose, manage, and treat these?

6. What is the best way to determine the differences in arter-ies between men and women, so we can discover the best treatments?

7. What is the best way to treat diastolic heart failure—normal heart function with abnormal heart relaxation—which is the most common type of heart failure in elderly women?

8. Why are young women more likely than men to die after suffer-ing a heart attack or after undergoing bypass surgery?

9. How do psychosocial issues such as stress, depression, and anx-iety impact women's hearts?

10. What are the most important heart disease risk factors for women, which lead to the worst outcomes, and how can we use this information to save women's lives?

It scares me that we don't know the answers to these questions yet, but I also want you to feel empowered because there is a lot we *do* know. I want to tell you what's going on out there. I want to let you in on some of the new, cutting-edge information. I want to tell you what might make a difference for your heart that your doctor might not know yet because it's not part of mainstream medical knowledge. Some of what I will share hasn't received its requisite seals of approval from every level of the scientific community. There are a lot of heart books out there that give you the textbook truths, but I want to give you the real-life truths, some of which are not conventional or found in those books.

Like I mentioned before, it can often take fifteen years for a research study to be executed and then published, so the gap between proof of a thought or hypothesis and publication for the public is really wide, let alone the gap between publication and new information being integrated into the standard of care. Then it's still advertised as a "new idea" or "new research" for a few more years. That means everything we know for sure about heart disease has been around for over a decade. It's old news.

But because I'm a cardiologist, I'm privy to a lot of information long before it hits the mainstream. I may not know everything, and the theories and studies I know about might not always turn out to be 100 percent right. Only time will tell. But I will never lead you toward anything harmful—I will only lead you toward what I sincerely believe, from my informed perspective, is going to help your heart.

I'm going to tell you what I know, and what the research is telling us right now—the tests that aren't always considered because they are not "gold standard" or haven't yet become standard of care, and the information that can affect how *you* decide to live your life. It's a lot more than you're going to hear in other books, a lot more than most doctors are going to be willing or even able to tell you. This book is filled with what we think we know right now, as well as an honest accounting of what we really don't know.

You can trust me. Nobody is giving me a grant to say anything, I'm not being funded, and I'm not trying to sell you any products. I am at liberty to be that voice that speaks the truth as I understand it. I'm giving you the gossip, the dirt on the street. I've scoured the science, taken notes from all my patients, and read, listened, watched, observed, seen the truth.

Choosing Your Fate

Wouldn't you want to know if the choices you're making today are affecting the length and quality of the rest of your life? Wouldn't you want to know if the stress you endure every day, the lack of sleep you tolerate, the huge amounts of caffeine you ingest, that glass of wine or vodka martini that you know is one drink too many, that decision to stay on the couch instead of to get up and exercise, that bag of chips or cookies, that overthinking and overstretching and overachieving and overdoing body and mind of yours, are literally, physically chipping away at the most central, life-sustaining organ in your body?

And if you knew it, would it change how you choose to live your life?

If I could tell you your future based on your present choices, wouldn't you want to know?

I've treated thousands of women in my office or met them through my work, and they are all examples of what can and will happen to the rest of us unless we change our behaviors, educate ourselves, and begin living our lives in a way that puts our hearts at the center.

Our choices catch up to us eventually. When we put on a seatbelt in a car, we think it's to prevent death in case of a crash, but we don't think about how it also might prevent us from hitting our heads, lacerating our faces, or being thrown from the car and breaking our legs. We think of the big final issues, but on the continuum of life, every decision we make could result in something other than we expect— age spots on our faces, scars that won't ever heal, bones that are never quite as strong as they were before they were broken, a heart that can't sustain us.

You are the one at risk. Yes, you, sitting right there, reading this book. I'm talking about the women who are struggling to maintain their status as commander-in-chief of their own lives and everyone else's around them. These are the women who are experiencing high blood pressure and high cholesterol and stress-induced inflammation and a prediabetic condition called metabolic syndrome, and these are all Heart Throbs that could indicate an increased chance of developing heart disease. These are the women having *heart attacks*. These are the women who think sleepless nights, stress, depression, anxiety, and hostility are "normal." These are the women who forget to take care of themselves first, and when they do remember, feel guilty about it.

Your heart is your most precious organ. It is the center of your universe. It fuels everything you do. If it stops beating, you stop living. It is indescribably important. It is practically synonymous with who you are and what you can do.

And yet we ignore our hearts. We can't see them, the way we can see our dimpled thighs or flabby upper arms. So we forget. We forget that with every beat, our hearts keep us alive. We forget that living in our heads builds up stress that literally puts too much pressure on our life source. We've forgotten how to live in a way that feeds us. We're starving.

You have a choice. You can go on doing what you are doing and risk it, hoping your heart will be okay. Or you can change, and feel better than you've felt in years, look better, enjoy your life more, and be pretty certain that you can protect your heart in the process too.

The Bottom Line

When I speak about women and heart disease prevention in public, I can see the fear in people's faces, and the quest for the truth. But when I tell people that 80 to 90 percent of heart disease cases are preventable, sometimes I'll see a woman roll her eyes. I've heard all the excuses: "I was born this way." "I'm big-boned." "Heart disease is in my family, so I'm going to get it no matter what." "I can't do anything about it."

That's just flat-out wrong! It's simply not true. Just as you can envision a future career, just as you can say, "Someday I want to do this," you can envision heart health, and you can also envision a healthier lifestyle. Then you can make it happen. Health is not something you have. It's something you go out and *get*.

This book is filled with the information you need to go in the right direction, to save your heart and yourself, because the truth is that you can't necessarily rely on your doctor to warn you, diagnose you, or treat you as effectively as he might warn, diagnose, or treat your father, your husband, your boyfriend, or your brother. More often than not, you are going to have to rely on yourself.

The next step is knowing what your risks are, and knowing what to do about it. So don't wait for a doctor to tell you what to do. You do it now. You save yourself.

Once you know what you need to do, please don't keep it to yourself. Share it with your mother, your sister, your best friends. They all need to understand that health—total health—begins in your heart. Your heart's job is not only to supply oxygen and nutrients to every corner of your body but to reflect how you live, how you think, how you love, and how you deal with life. The studies that show the benefits of laughter on the heart and that demonstrate the negative role of anger and hostility are the same studies that, in fine print, are reminding us that the heart is literally, metaphorically, and spiritually the center of what makes us who we are. How we choose to live affects this epicenter, and this reverberates into every other aspect of our lives.

If we put our hearts at the center of our lives, then the ripple effect will be health, vitality, happiness, love, and longevity. Making a healthy heart is not just about dieting and exercising. It is also about an awareness of the effects of joy, stress, laughter, relaxation, anxiety, hostility, depression, control, and love. They all affect your heart. If women don't understand that heart disease prevention is an active choice, then they relinquish the opportunity to live longer, healthier, stronger, and better lives.

So be honest with yourself. Understand who you are. And then commit to a life living from the heart. Once you have a handle on that, the rest is easy.

Let's grab a hold of that handle together.

This Chapter, by Heart

♥ Heart disease is the number-one killer of women.

♥ Heart disease is preventable.

♥ Modern medicine hasn't caught up with women's heart health yet, so your doctor may not recognize signs of heart disease in you.

♥ Your heart reflects every aspect of your health and life.

♥ Ultimately, you are the most qualified person to heal your own heart. The future of your heart, your health, and your life is in your own hands.

CHAPTER TWO

Heart Throbs: Beyond Risk Factors

Your heart beats again, and again, and again, multiple times each minute, for hours, days, weeks, years. Right there in the middle of your chest, it is beating, keeping you alive with each pulse. Every breath, every thought, every step, everything you do depends on it. It is the essence of you. So let's talk about it. How have you been treating your heart?

We take our hearts for granted to such an extent that I don't think most women realize that they could even be at risk for heart disease. In 2011, a survey was done on a large group of women, asking them whether they knew heart disease was the number-one killer of women. In this particular survey, 90 percent said yes, they knew this. Great, right? These results sound optimistic.

But here's the part that bothered me. When each of those same women were asked whether heart disease was *her* problem, only 13 percent said yes.

This is exactly the kind of information that drives me crazy and keeps me up all night.

There is a huge disconnect here. We know *the* risk, but we don't know *our* risk, and that's why we don't take it seriously. We think heart disease is somebody else's problem . . . until it happens to us.

Here's the thing that every woman needs to realize today: When you have heart disease, it starts decades before you get sick. Heart disease could be gearing up in your arteries, changing the course of your life. And here's the kicker: Decades before that heart attack, you could have been doing things to change the course of your life.

I'm talking about *right now*. You are at that "decades before" place, or even nearer. This is the moment. Even if you are postmenopausal and at greater risk, it's not too late to prevent it from happening. We know more than we think we know about the state of our own bodies. You *know* when you aren't feeling well. You *know* when you aren't taking care of yourself. You *know* when you are out of balance, when you are going in a bad direction, when you've been physically or emotionally hurt, when you are too stressed out to sleep or think straight.

And you know that heart disease is the number-one killer of women.

It's time to connect the dots.

Because you need to know, really know, in the way that makes you want to do something about it, that the stress and pain and heartache and poor dietary choices and sedentary lifestyle and cigarettes and bottles of wine and job fretting and relationship self-torture and parental anxiety and all the other things you do every day that you *know* aren't good for you are hurting your heart *now*. They are contributing to your future heart attack *today*. We might not call this "heart disease" in the medical world, but guess what? You are already heart sick.

In this chapter, I want to make you aware of your risks, no matter how young you are and no matter how healthy you feel right now, so you can determine whether *now*, rather than later, is the time to make some changes. Heart disease is not just about developing plaque in the arteries. It starts from a place of being unwell, of not being true to yourself. It starts by failing to give your heart, and by extension your whole self, what it needs.

Traditionally, doctors talk about risk factors for heart disease, and public health studies have focused on finding and measuring risk factors in the general population, such as high blood pressure, high cholesterol, and smoking. All that can be helpful, but the problem I see is that a lot of these so-called risk factors are already major signs of heartsickness. When you have high cholesterol, that isn't a sign that you might get sick. It's a sign that *you are already sick*. The idea of a "risk factor" makes it sound like something that could someday lead to a problem. No. The risk factor *is part of the problem*, so let's rename the term right this minute.

Instead of talking about risk factors, I want to talk about Heart Throbs. Not the kind your preteen daughter swoons over, but the throb in your metaphorical heart that gets your attention and signals an imbalance in your heart and, by extension, your life. A Heart Throb, the way I use the term, is a measure of your vitality, of your heart and mind, of your very life. I want you to feel yours. Know yours. And understand what they mean, not in the context of a study or a research trial or the last article your doctor read in a medical journal, but in the context of *you*.

To understand how important these Heart Throbs are to your life and health, I want to get a little technical. Bear with me, because this is about you and what's inside your body, and it's something I believe you absolutely must understand if the term *Heart Throb* is going to mean anything to you. I want to introduce you to your *endothelium*.

We all have pocketbooks to carry our stuff. You've got the leather on the outside, and the lining on the inside. Now think about what happens when you get a little tear or cut in the lining of your purse. All of a sudden, you can't find your keys, your gum, your lipstick, your wallet, the kitchen sink. You start digging through your purse and then suddenly you see it: that fateful tear. All the things you need have slipped through and are floating around between the leather and the lining of your pocketbook.

Your arteries have a lining too, and it's called the *endothelium*. There's a lot of medical talk in the media, but it isn't often about the endothelium. It's not a glamorous topic. It's like talking about the lining of your purse. Who cares about the lining of your purse? The color, the shape, the style of your purse—now, those are fun topics. And what's in a woman's purse? Fascinating. But the lining? Boring! However, boring as it may seem, the endothelium affects your health in a broad and significant way.

The endothelium is a lot like the lining of a purse. But your endothelium lines every artery in your entire body, from your brain to your big toe. It goes everywhere, in and out of your heart and up and down. A healthy endothelium means every part of your body is getting the nutrients it needs, and that the arteries are functioning the way they should, relaxing and contracting normally. But when things go wrong, endothelial dysfunction can manifest anywhere, not just in the heart. It's a system-wide issue.

You can't see endothelial dysfunction. You can't feel it, but the endothelium can get those little cuts and tears, just like the lining of your purse, from all kinds of things you do to yourself. Smoking, processed foods, inflammation related to obesity, and a sedentary lifestyle can all result in the endothelium getting stiff and losing its elasticity. When that happens, the lining can develop micro-tears from all the poor lifestyle choices. Once the endothelium has been compromised, stuff starts to slip through—stuff like cholesterol and oxidized LDL, collagen, and smooth muscle cells. You don't necessarily need to know what they all are, but you should know that they do not belong where they are going, lodged between the lining and the artery wall. This causes an immune response in the artery as it tries to fight off these things it detects as foreign invaders, sending other cells called macrophages to defend it. The artery wall is no longer protected. It gets inflamed, like your skin around a splinter. It gets bumpy and starts snagging chunks of fat. It gets clogged. This is how the scary clogged arteries you hear so much about get started. Suddenly, that expensive purse you bought is worthless because whenever you use it, you know you won't be able to find your keys.

A damaged endothelium is bad news for your heart, and it's bad news for the rest of you too. Remember, your arteries go everywhere in your body. So overall, healthy arteries mean health, and damaged arteries mean illness. A healthy endothelium can prevent that cascade of events that leads to some of those Heart Throbs that can trigger heart disease and so many other chronic problems.

So why aren't we more invested in keeping our endothelium healthy? I can tell you this: You can eliminate many of your own Heart Throbs—those things that cut and tear and ravage your endothelium. You can pay attention to your Heart Throbs, and you can modify them so they aren't throbbing in your life anymore. The health of your arteries is *up to you*. Sometimes we are nicer to our favorite pocketbook than we are to our own hearts.

Your Heart Throbs

For years, I've been looking at lifestyle factors, or Heart Throbs, in women and also in men that can compromise the integrity of the endothelium. Heart Throbs determine the level of wellness and vitality in an individual patient. Let's look at these together to determine how your endothelium is likely doing.

This is your long, hard look in the mirror. These are the things that don't just push you toward heartsickness but can put you at risk for illness in every form, from cancer, dementia, liver failure, and aging to depression, anxiety, and unhappiness. When these Heart Throbs are off, they will sap your vitality, throw you out of balance, and destroy the linings of your arteries, from your heart to your kidneys to your brain.

Remember, you are taking responsibility for your own health now. I'm not giving you this information so you can form some vague theoretical concept of "healthy." I'm giving you this information so you can discover precisely how the way you are living your life now is affecting your heart, your organs, and your vitality. I will tell you the public health perspective, because that is how we help motivate change, but when you read this list, take it personally. I'm not talking about "people." I'm talking about *you*.

Some of the Heart Throbs listed here are standard risk factors cardiologists would consider in a heart disease patient, but the way I am using this term is specifically to define *your* individual lifestyle and where you personally (rather than you as a public health statistic) might be living in a way that could hurt your heart. Let's figure out exactly where you stand. After reading each section, check the Heart Throb that you think applies to you.

Dr. Steinbaum's Heart Throbs

YOUR EXERCISE TOLERANCE

The first Heart Throb I want you to think seriously about it this: How easily can you exercise? Exercise is the most potent and powerful medicine known to humankind. Movement equals life. Movement is a sign of vitality. If you can't walk a couple of blocks or if you can't climb two flights of stairs (or if you fail a stress test—more about that in Chapter 8), then I guarantee you are at risk for heart disease.

Someone who is physically in great shape has a heart that doesn't have to work as hard to perform an activity. For example, a marathon runner has a resting heart rate that is very low. When she starts running, her heart rate might go up, but slowly and to an optimal level to deliver oxygen for the amount of work that the body is performing. A sedentary person, on the other hand, may have a heart that has to labor dramatically just to get her up the stairs. When you can't get on a treadmill and walk briskly for at least four minutes, you are really out of shape.

This doesn't happen out of nowhere. It is not an accident when you are unable to sustain exercise. You probably spend most of your time sitting—in the car, at a desk, on the couch. It's not genetic. Bodies naturally want to move, and it takes some effort to habitually stop moving your body. But when not moving becomes your new habit, as you age, it will take more and more effort to stay vital.

There was a lot of buzz in the media recently about a study that looked at the number of hours people sat each day, and how that correlated to their risk of death from all causes. Those who sat for more than eleven hours a day had the highest risk of death. Second in line were those who sat between eight and eleven hours per day. Those who sat for fewer than four hours a day had the lowest risk of death from all causes. This study looked at over 200,000 people for three years, and the result was clear: The more you sit, the more you are at risk. So what kind of life are you living? If you go from your bed to your car to your desk to your car to your couch in front of the TV and then back to bed every day, you are more likely to be obese, to have diabetes, to develop dementia, and, of course, to have heart disease. And if you don't have any of those things yet, you are more likely to find them in your future. This is the most important thing I want you to remember: A sedentary life can transform you from someone who doesn't *like* to exercise into someone who *can't* exercise before you even realize it's happening, and that's not just the beginning of the end. That's merely a couple of shaky steps from the end.

YOUR RESTING HEART RATE

How fast your heart beats while you are resting is directly related to how fit your heart is. Hearts tend to get more pliable with exercise, which means that they do a better job of filling up with blood and sending it throughout the body. The heart, like the arteries, needs to be relaxed and able to passively fill with blood, like a balloon. Hearts that beat less are more efficient at this process. Hearts that are stiff, or sick, need to beat more to deliver the same amount of blood because they can't fill up as well. That's why people who get more exercise tend to have a lower resting heart rate and people who are sedentary tend to have a higher resting heart rate. Because a high resting heart rate puts you at greater risk for heart disease, and because you can change your resting heart rate by moving more, you should know what yours is, and then work on improving it if it is too high.

The best time to take your resting heart rate is right after you wake up in the morning, before you get out of bed. Find your pulse at your wrist or neck and count it for fifteen seconds, then multiply that number times four.

My opinion of what constitutes a high resting heart rate is a little stricter than the one generally accepted by doctors, because resting heart rate directly correlates to exercise and how the body's nervous system is wired. Traditionally, a resting heart rate was considered too high if it was over 100 beats per minute (BPM), but I say it's too high if it's over 70. If your heart rate is 70 to 90 beats per minute at rest, then your heart is working too hard. The most perfect resting heart rate, in my opinion, is between 50 and 70 beats per minute. A marathon runner might reach a heart rate of 90 well into a run, but his or her resting heart rate may be as low as 40.

Heart rate recovery time, or how fast your heartbeat returns to baseline after you exercise, also tells you what kind of shape you are in. After a stress test, I always like to see how long it takes to go below 100 beats per minute. If it is less than a minute, then you are in pretty good shape.

Heart Beats

A Women's Health Initiative study of more than 100,000 women showed that a heart rate greater than 76 BPM was associated with a 26 percent increased risk of heart attack in the following 7.8 years, compared to one that's less than 62 BPM. This relationship between resting pulse and risk of heart events was strongest in postmenopausal women between the ages of 50 and 64 years old. Physical activity is the key element in preventing a high resting heart rate in women of all ages.

YOUR HEART RATE VARIABILITY

This Heart Throb reflects your heart's physiologic state. Heart rate variability is governed by your autonomic nervous system, which controls many functions in the body—heart rate, digestion, breathing, sweating, salivating, sexual arousal—without you having to worry about them. After the endothelium, the autonomic nervous system is the true keeper of our hearts. It decides whether one of two subsystems are running the show at any given time. These two subsystems are the "fight or flight" system and the "rest and digest" system. When you are stressed or out of shape, the fight-or-flight system, or sympathetic system, takes over. The resting nervous system, or the parasympathetic nervous system, keeps things calm, the heart rate slow, and is a sign of a well-oiled machine.

When your heart is calm and healthy, and when the parasympathetic system is running things, there is a beat-to-beat variation in the heart rate, affected by breathing. When you are out of shape, or the adrenal, anxiety-ridden sympathetic system is in overdrive, your heart rate variability decreases. This could be one of the first signs that your cardiovascular system may not be fit.

You can measure your own heart rate variability with this test: Find your pulse in your wrist or neck. Now, take a deep, slow breath in to the count of four, and then a deep, slow breath out to the count of six. Exhale fully and completely. If you can feel your heart rate slowing down slightly with your exhalation, that means you have good vagal tone. In other words, your parasympathetic nervous system has turned on and is slowing things down based on the signal that slow breathing sends to your brain: that everything is working efficiently. You passed the test!

This exercise can be difficult for some people, so if you aren't sure, or you start hyperventilating just trying to find your pulse, use a heart rate monitor. I suggest investing in one, anyway, so you can keep track of your heart rate while you exercise. Then try this again, being sure to take a very deep slow breath in. When you exhale fully, watch the monitor to see if your heart rate slows down.

Doing this small test can really demonstrate the power of breathing. It also demonstrates just who's in control: your head or your heart. If your heart rate doesn't slow down when you do this (try it a few times to be sure), you may have low heart rate variability.

This can mean several different things. If your head has taken over and is counting beats per minute and is totally convinced something must be terribly wrong, causing you to freak out and hyperventilate, you may be getting a false reading. Or you might be so out of shape that not even deep breathing can change your heart rate.

In either of these cases, your body is waving a red flag, hoping you'll take notice, because something has got to change. Start with taking a deep breath, then plan your exercise strategy. Both of those will turn on the vagal tone and put the autonomic nervous system back in control.

YOUR SMOKING HABIT

If you smoke cigarettes, you don't need me to tell you that it's bad for your health, and you probably already know you are at greater risk for lung cancer. You might also know that smoking cigarettes is the most common preventable cause of death on the planet. But did you know it also put you at major risk for heart disease?

If you smoke, you might avoid lung cancer, but those cigarettes are doing serious damage to your endothelium. With every inhalation of toxic smoke, you are flooding your body with chemicals that can damage your endothelium, causing little cuts and tears that will eventually lead to hardened arteries that cannot flex, expand, and contract.

The chemicals you inhale from smoking also force your blood vessels to contract, increasing your blood pressure and your risk of developing a blood clot. The chemicals in cigarette smoke can also cause plaque ruptures, which can lead to a sudden heart attack. Also, people who smoke tend to have lower levels of HDL (good) cholesterol. When young people are wheeled into the emergency room because of a heart attack, nine times out of ten, cigarettes had something to do with it. Every inhalation is like a round of Russian Roulette, putting you at risk at that very moment. Oddly enough, I always see blockages in the top part of the main artery of the heart in smokers, which is the artery that if blocked could possibly kill you. Those cigarettes don't mess around. Their damage tends to go right to the worst spots.

So if you smoke, this is your likely future: dropping dead of a heart attack, maybe today, maybe tomorrow, maybe in a few years. You never know which drag might actually be the one that does you in. I know I'm being dramatic, but I'm also telling the truth. There is no such thing as "safe smoking." You can't put a condom on a cigarette.

I know it's hard to give up smoking. I do. I get annoyed when I see those health lists that say, "Quit smoking," as if it's nothing, as if all you have to do is put down your cigarette and say, "Okay, I guess I won't do that anymore." I get it. I'm not going to blow smoke at you and tell you it's easy.

But we're talking about your life here. We're talking about your heart. If you smoke just one to three cigarettes a day, if you only bum a cigarette off your friends at happy hour after work, you are at greater risk for a heart attack, not to mention a stroke, cancer, and a bunch of other unpleasant diseases you'd probably rather not even know about, like peripheral vascular disease and COPD. And if you use birth control pills and smoke a pack of cigarettes a day, your risk of having a heart attack goes up thirtyfold. Yes, we all have the freedom to make choices, but I've never met a smoker who didn't feel tied to her cigarettes. I wouldn't call that freedom. I would call that a dangerous game that you're going to lose. And if all that won't convince you, then maybe this will: Smoking causes wrinkles! If I can't appeal to your health, perhaps I can appeal to your vanity.

But the minute you stop smoking is the minute your body begins fixing itself.

If you don't smoke, never do it. If you do smoke, you've simply got to find a way to stop, and the sooner, the better. There are many ways to get help quitting smoking. Ask your doctor about it. Make an appointment today. Get the patch or take medication to ease yourself off the poison. Get whatever help you need. Do it for your life. Pretty please.

YOUR CHOLESTEROL LEVEL

Your cholesterol level may not seem like the first thing on your list of health concerns. High cholesterol is that problem your grandfather has, right? Or maybe your father? You don't even eat red meat! Actually, it could be your problem too. In women patients, the most common Heart Throb is lipid abnormalities—in other words, high LDL (bad) cholesterol, low HDL (good) cholesterol, or high triglycerides. I'll tell you all about cholesterol tests in Chapter 8, but for now, suffice it to say that you should know your overall cholesterol number, as well as your LDL (bad) and HDL (good) cholesterol levels and triglycerides. Younger and younger people are finding they have high cholesterol, mostly because of a poor diet, but in some cases because of genetics. Your total cholesterol should be under 200. If your LDL is above 130, you are 2.2 times more likely to develop heart disease than someone with normal cholesterol. If it's above 160, you are three times more likely to develop heart disease. HDL levels should be above 40 for men and above 50 for women, but above 60 is highly protective against heart disease, so that's what I like to see.

Heart Sense

My patients often forget which cholesterol is the "good" one and which cholesterol is the "bad" one. This is the way I remember: LDL is the "bad" one because L stands for "the Lower, the better," or "Lousy." HDL is the "good" one because H stands for "the Higher, the better," or "Happy."

HDL cholesterol is important. It is a potent anti-inflammatory, prevents clots, inhibits oxidation, and keeps the endothelium of the arteries protected from that LDL that leads to plaque formation. I think of it like that '80s computer game Pac-Man, eating the little dots of cholesterol, or at least shuttling the bad cholesterol out of the arteries. HDL is often high in younger women who have estrogen, which is one of the reasons young women aren't assumed to be at risk for heart disease. However, HDL decreases with age and the decrease in estrogen that goes along with menopause.

HDL comes in many different particle sizes. The HDL2b is a big, fluffy HDL that is capable of carrying out the cholesterol-laden LDL particles. This is the most effective HDL and is directly related to estrogen and to exercise. As a woman gets older and her estrogen decreases, so does her HDL, unless she exercises. When I see low HDL2bs, I know that person is not exercising enough.

While writing this book, I took a course on cutting-edge information in cardiology. One of the world-renowned researchers in cholesterol, lipids, and plaque development stated that just the week before, they'd discovered that all HDLs are the same, and that, in fact, these HDL2bs are not any better than the other kinds, as we previously believed. He said that all HDL particle sizes work the same.

After my mouth dropped to the floor, I thought that I needed to edit this chapter ASAP! But then I thought about how quickly information is evolving in the field of cardiology, and how much we still don't know. As of today, the HDL theory has been dispelled, but I can tell you that with my patients in my office, this HDL2b marker continues to correlate to my patients' exercise regimes. I can tell right away if someone hasn't been exercising simply from this marker. It is almost like I have been spying on them!

We will continue to wait for the research to solve some of these unanswered questions, but the reality is that no matter what, the higher the HDL is, the more protective it is to your arteries. For every 1 mg/dl drop in HDL, there is a 3 to 4 percent increased risk in women, and a 2 to 3 percent increased risk in men, of developing heart disease. Sometimes a low HDL is genetic, and I see a trend from fathers to sons passing along this low HDL, and sometimes to daughters too. This significantly increases the risk of heart disease. In fact, in women, this trend is more significant to the development of premature plaque in the arteries.

LDL also comes in different particle sizes, and although LDL is traditionally the most implicated player in the development of arterial plaque, we know that alone, that number doesn't give us the whole risk picture. You have to consider particle size. There are some LDLs that aren't as destructive as others. These are the bigger, "fluffier" particle sizes. The smaller, denser sizes do more damage. They are completely filled with cholesterol, and these are the plaque generators.

Their protein helpers are also critical risk markers. You know that oil and water don't mix. When an LDL particle is densely filled with cholesterol, it is oily, and that kind of oil can't go through the bloodstream because the blood is largely made of water. It needs a carrier, something that can move through the blood vessels, shuttling the LDL particle where it needs to go. This carrier is the apolipoprotein B, a protein that transports these cholesterol-filled LDL through the bloodstream. When you have high numbers of this protein, it tells us that there are high numbers of plaque-forming, cholesterol-filled particles that are headed right to the arteries, where they will deposit plaque. Because the lighter, fluffier LDL particles don't require this assistance, your apolipoprotein B number is highly correlated to plaque deposits, especially in women. Every LDL with an apolipoprotein B is a plaque builder. Apolipoprotein B numbers vary according to the lab that runs the test. For the most common test, your number should be below 80 mg/dl, but ask your doctor what your number should be. (I'll talk more about lipid tests in Chapter 8.)

Lp(a) is a protein that attaches to LDL, causing the blood to clot more easily. This also increases your risk of heart disease and stroke. This is a genetic marker, passed down from generation to generation, and is often associated with premature plaque and heart disease in young people. In fact, when I see young people who have a family history of heart disease, and a normal cholesterol with plaque in the arteries, usually I find this sneaky protein behind the scenes. Unfortunately, this is one of the few Heart Throbs for which diet and exercise do not make a difference. You can be as healthy as can be and still have this problem. Because this trait is passed down, it's good to know your family history. If you have a family history of heart disease, then you should definitely get this one checked. The only way to treat it is with a long-acting B-complex derivative called niacin.

Last, triglycerides are also part of the cholesterol profile, and high triglyceride levels are associated with eating too many carbohydrates and sugars. In women, high triglycerides are a more potent risk for heart disease than they are in men, so you really want to keep track of this number and keep it in the normal range, which is less than 150 mg/dl. The good news is that this one is easily correctable through lifestyle changes.

If you are a young woman without any obvious risk factors according to the established standard of care doctors use, your doctor might not test your cholesterol unless you ask. Ask, because high cholesterol is a major Heart Throb for women, and everybody knows it, and has known it for decades. Being a young woman does not make you immune, and the bottom line is that your doctor can't *see* high cholesterol. He can't know you have it unless he tests you for it.

For a few people, medication to control cholesterol is necessary, but for most of us, all we have to do is improve what we eat and how much we move and our cholesterol levels will normalize pretty quickly. You have the power.

YOUR BLOOD PRESSURE

Blood pressure is another thing young women don't think they need to pay attention to unless they get sick, but high blood pressure is more common than you might think. One in three adults has high blood pressure. That's 65 million Americans! They call high blood pressure the "silent killer" because 30 percent of those with high blood pressure don't even know they have it. You might be one of them.

Everyone, at any age, should know and monitor blood pressure, and not just once a year, because it can change from moment to moment depending on what's going on in your life. The only way to get an accurate blood pressure is to take an average over several readings. If it is borderline high in the doctor's office, you might want to recheck it again in a month or so, just to be sure that it is not headed in the upward direction. Just go to the doctor and put your arm out. They'll do a blood pressure check. Or go to the local pharmacy and stick your arm into one of those sleeves. Then you'll know whether this is one of your areas of concern or whether you don't have to worry about it for now.

Blood pressure consists of two numbers: a top number, called systolic, and a bottom number, called diastolic. The systolic blood pressure is the pressure against your arteries when your heart is pumping. The diastolic blood pressure is the pressure against your arteries when your heart is at rest, between pumps, when the heart is meant to fill with blood. Traditional risk assessment criteria only looked at the systolic blood pressure, but high diastolic pressure is dangerous too. If that number is high, that means your heart or your arteries can't relax. That could mean your endothelium is already getting stiff. There is no gentle passive filling of blood, and that's a definite warning sign. It is the beginning of a process that results in plaque developing in the arteries. Sometimes blood pressure increases for other reasons besides age. It can increase as a result of medications, such as oral contraceptives, decongestants, or some others.

Normal blood pressure is less than 120/80 mm Hg. Borderline high blood pressure or "prehypertension" is blood pressure between 120/80 to 139/89. Once you get to 140/90, you officially have high blood pressure, and that is one of the major and well-understood risks for heart disease. A healthy artery relaxes. An artery under high pressure is an artery that's forcing your heart to work too hard. If you are diabetic or have multiple Heart Throbs including high blood pressure, you should take medication, because you don't want to just "wait out" high blood pressure, especially in these situations. Even lifestyle changes may not work quickly enough (although they will certainly help lower your blood pressure).

Blood pressure, like many of the Heart Throbs, increases with age. My patients often say, "I never had high blood pressure before." I say, "You were never fifty before." Unfortunately, it's the direction our bodies take, unless we fight against the body's tendency to do this.

But you can start training for this, before you ever get high blood pressure. If half of 60-year-olds have high blood pressure, that means half don't. Which side do you want to fall into when you turn 60? Practicing good dietary and exercise habits, cutting down on salt, keeping your weight under control, and managing your stress (stress has a huge impact on blood pressure) are what you should be practicing now to avoid high blood pressure later. Even if you already have high blood pressure and you are on medication for it, these lifestyle strategies are absolutely crucial if you want to preserve your vitality. Your blood pressure number doesn't exist in a vacuum. It's a marker that says something about your total well-being. If you start changing your habits now, you can change your outcome. You might even be able to go off those pills, with your doctor's approval. I mean it. Taking pills is not a life sentence. You can likely come off them when your lifestyle changes.

YOUR BLOOD SUGAR, METABOLIC SYNDROME, OR DIABETES

Imagine the inside of a watch, with all those tiny, precise cog wheels. Now imagine pouring honey all over it—sticky, sugary honey. Now how well do you think that watch is going to work?

Diabetes is a serious, life-threatening disease in which your blood sugar and insulin system no longer work because you have more sugar coming in than your body can handle. This messes with your entire system in many dangerous ways. It is destructive to all your arteries and your organs, it puts you at risk for a heart attack, and it lowers the quality of your life.

While some people are born with type 1 diabetes and don't have the body chemistry to metabolize sugar, the biggest population and lifestyle problem is type 2 diabetes. This is a group of diseases marked by high levels of sugar in the bloodstream, due to the body's inability to properly metabolize sugar.

Diabetes affects 25.8 million people in the U.S., 7 million of whom don't even know they have it. Your risk of having diabetes increases with age: 26.9 percent of all people 65 years or older have diabetes. Plus, 79 million more have a prediabetic condition called metabolic syndrome, which means they are likely to get diabetes soon if they keep doing what they are doing.

Metabolic syndrome is associated with blood sugars greater than 100, blood pressure greater than 130/85, a waist circumference of greater than 35 inches for women and 40 inches for men, an HDL less than 50 mg/dl for women and less than 40 mg/dl for men, and triglycerides greater than 150 mg/dl. The diagnosis is made if you have three or more of these factors.

Initially, what happens when diabetes is developing is a desensitization of the body's ability to maintain blood sugar at normal levels. In a healthy person, when sugar enters the bloodstream, insulin is released to break it down. When the body is overwhelmed by sugars, this mechanism is slowed and becomes ineffective, so more insulin is required than normal to bring the sugar levels down. This leads to high insulin levels and borderline high sugar levels, as the insulin is increasingly unable to do its job. As this process worsens, the sugar becomes more resistant to coming down, the insulin goes through the roof, and eventually, your body loses all ability to regulate sugars and insulin, resulting in what we call type 2 diabetes. Type 2 diabetes can lead to many other health issues, including heart attacks, kidney disease, strokes, peripheral vascular disease, blindness, neuropathy, gastrointestinal issues, and infections—basically, it wreaks havoc in every organ system in the body.

Diabetes causes a lot of serious health problems, but what a lot of people may not know is that diabetes is a major Heart Throb for heart disease. In fact, if you have diabetes, you are just as likely to have a heart attack as someone who has already had a heart attack. This is called a coronary artery disease risk equivalent. The risk is even worse for women than men—seven times worse. The longer you have diabetes, the higher the chance that you are going to die from it, and the higher the chance that your death will be from a heart attack (although it might also be kidney failure or an infection, and those are no fun, either).

The reality is that this can all be controlled with a low-carbohydrate and low-sugar diet, weight loss, and exercise. It's not easy, but it's not mysterious. You can control whether you develop this condition by what you choose to do. This is, simply put, a lifestyle disease. Look down. If you can't see your feet because your belly is in the way, you know you'd better do something, and quickly.

If you think you might be one of those people who has diabetes, or metabolic syndrome, but doesn't know it, please find out! Call your doctor today. You need a fasting blood sugar test and/or a hemoglobin A1C test. Your fasting blood sugar should be less than 100. The HbA1C is a more specific test, telling you an average of your blood sugars over three months' time, to give you an idea of how efficiently your body is processing all that sugar you eat.

Every day you have diabetes and don't do something about it puts you at greater risk. It doesn't make sense to hide your head in the sand. You need to *know the truth*. You need to find out if this is you.

Because the power to change it is in your hands. All the lifestyle changes I talk about in this book will decrease your chance of developing diabetes, and can even reverse the disease, but the most important ones are limiting sugar and simple starches like foods made from white flour; never, ever, ever drinking sodas or sugar-sweetened beverages (never!); losing excess weight; and exercising regularly. (Even diet sodas have been shown to contribute to this problem, so just stop. Remember water?)

YOUR INFLAMMATION

Now let's talk about something a little less obvious than your weight or what's on your dinner plate or in your wine glass. Let's talk about something you can't see at all but that is wreaking havoc inside your body: inflammation.

Inflammation is the new buzzword in cardiology these days, because more doctors are beginning to believe that inflammation is a key contributor to heart disease, and that it has been previously overlooked, especially in women. We also know that inflammation contributes to the plaque ruptures that can cause unexpected heart attacks. One study showed that particularly in women, inflammation may more accurately predict who will have heart disease than a high LDL ("bad") cholesterol level alone. Your level of inflammation is measured by a blood test called high-sensitivity C-reactive protein, which indicates the level of inflammation in the arteries. This wasn't something previous risk-analysis methods ever looked at. When this risk factor was added to the analysis, many of the women who were *not* supposedly at risk were suddenly at risk after all.

Remember your endothelium? Those cuts and tears you are trying to avoid can cause cholesterol to slip into your arteries. This leads to inflammation because inflammatory cells try to fight off the "foreign" cholesterol "invaders." This process compromises the arteries' flexibility and strength, increasing the possibility of further arterial damage—more cuts and tears—and more ports of entry for cholesterol and other foreign junk that isn't supposed to be there. This leads to plaque formation, especially if there is no treatment for Heart Throbs, and this arterial plaque greatly increases your risk of heart attack. It's a vicious cycle, and inflammation is just a part of it, but if you do have inflammation, it is a sign that this process is happening in your arteries.

Inflammation can also be caused by other issues, like infection or autoimmune disease, but inflammation in the arteries is the most dangerous kind when it comes to heart health. For many people, an elevated inflammatory marker is probably caused by health-compromising factors like smoking, a poor diet, stress, and excess body fat, particularly belly fat.

One common way your doctor can determine whether or not you have inflammation is through the high-sensitivity C-reactive protein test, or hs-CRP test. I'll talk more about this test in Chapter 8.

YOUR APOE GENES

Genetics can influence your heart disease risk in many ways, and one of the ways I find incredibly interesting and instructive is the ApoE genotype. Although not all doctors know about or think this gene is relevant to heart health, I find it is particularly helpful for dietary guidance.

Your apolipoprotein E (ApoE) gene is a gene on chromosome 19 that indicates certain disease susceptibility and is also correlated with the body's ability to metabolize certain kinds of foods. If you have one or two ApoE-2 or ApoE-4 genes, you are at greater risk for heart disease, among other health conditions, and you will not metabolize all foods as well as someone with the more common ApoE-3 gene would. Specifically, if you have one or two of the ApoE-2 genes, your body cannot tolerate sugars or simple carbohydrates. Starch, simple carbohydrates, and sugar tend to cause high triglycerides in these people. If you have one or two of the ApoE-4 genes, you'll have a harder time managing fats. Meat, dairy, and fatty foods tend to contribute to very high LDL cholesterol and arterial plaque, and I usually recommend that people with this problem eat a vegetarian, vegan, or at least extremely low-fat diet. Many people with early plaque development are APO 3/4 or 4/4 and should never eat saturated fats. I'll talk more about how to get tested to determine your ApoE gene in Chapter 8.

YOUR HORMONAL ISSUES

Girls, this Heart Throb is for you in particular, although the men in your lives might want to keep reading just for the sake of enlightenment. I'm seeing more and more hormonal issues in my patients these days. This includes women who battle serious premenstrual or menopausal symptoms, and women who are surprised to discover they are infertile. I believe that a woman's hormonal cycle is like the canary in the coal mine. It's often the first hint that something is going wrong at a system-wide level.

Women who have hormonal issues, including health issues during pregnancy like elevations in sugar or high blood pressure, or who experience early menopause, are more likely to develop heart disease later in life. Keeping track of your hormonal issues, including your menstrual cycles, pregnancies, miscarriages, and menopause, can help you and your doctor determine your risk. Hormonal imbalance is a Heart Throb that doctors don't always consider.

As we go through menopause, the natural decline in estrogen is normal, but until we get there, we should have a steady amount that fluctuates according to the menstrual cycle. If you have any sort of hormonal issue, consider it a warning to pay closer attention to your heart health and to your other Heart Throbs. Hormonal issues could be what tip the scale. I'll talk more about hormonal issues later, but for now, keep it on your radar.

YOUR FAMILY HISTORY

Enough of the tests and numbers. Now I want to move into some other areas that are just as crucial to understand in terms of your risk of developing heart disease. One of the big ones is family history.

The traditional risk factor analysis looks for heart disease in your father before age 55, and in your mother before age 65, or in either parent before age 60. But this is not the end of the story when it comes to heart disease. At least not in my book.

Forget the numbers. Just look at your family. Causes of death often run in families. In some families, you see a lot of cancer. In others, you see a lot of heart disease, even if it happens to most family members over age 60. Maybe it's not a parent. Maybe it's an aunt or an uncle, or several grandparents, or even worse, a sibling, which definitely puts you at risk.

I've also had patients whose parents didn't die of a heart attack until after age 60, but then I find out, when I ask more questions, that many of them suffered from strokes, angina, mild heart attacks, or acute coronary syndromes (more about what all these are later in this book) before they ever had a massive or fatal heart attack. Those count too. If you don't know your family history, you need to ask anybody who might know, if that's possible, because family history is definitely a predictor of heart disease risk.

If Great-Aunt Stephanie or Grandpa Harvey or Cousin Joshua died at 45 and you don't know why, find out why. Maybe nobody talked about causes of death back then, but the information matters to you now. If several family members, no matter what age, died of heart disease, you are at risk, and the way you choose to live your life is even more crucial to your health and survival.

And by the way, even if your family's history is riddled with the C-word (cancer) but nobody ever gets heart disease, you can still develop it by living a heart-wrecking lifestyle. Nobody is immune.

YOUR BODY FAT

I bet you've been waiting for me to talk about your weight. Of course I will, because over half of Americans are overweight, with a full 30 percent of those people qualifying as obese. Most people carry too much weight around, and that puts an immense strain on your heart, your other internal organs, your ability to exercise, even your ability to feel comfortable sitting in a chair. It also puts you at risk for so many other health problems, including diabetes, high cholesterol, high blood pressure, and many of the other Heart Throbs. Get fat, get diabetes, then get heart disease. It doesn't matter what order you pile on the Heart Throbs. They all come to the same thing in the end.

Abdominal obesity in particular is risky because the fat on your belly behaves differently than fat in other parts of your body, triggering the release of a slew of hormones and chemicals that are associated with heart disease. Excess abdominal fat in particular has been linked to higher triglycerides, prediabetes, and inflammation. Look at yourself in the mirror. Where do you carry your excess weight? Believe it or not, if it is in your butt, you are much better off, so try not to complain too much!

I'm going to talk about weight a lot in this book, because I think it's the thing people struggle with the most but that they are most able to control. It's also the catalyst for so many other Heart Throbs. If you manage your weight, you are much less likely to get high cholesterol, high blood pressure, or diabetes. It's like knocking out four Heart Throbs in one.

A lot of my patients tell me they can't lose weight because being overweight runs in their families, but recent research is proving how much control we have over our so-called genetic destinies. It's true that people with overweight or obese parents are more likely to be overweight or obese as adults, but it is not a rule. You're just as likely to "inherit" lifestyle habits you can change. What you do influences how genes get turned on or off, and that's a more powerful indicator of body weight than the weight of your parents.

I believe the best way to gauge your weight is by using the Body Mass Index, or BMI. This is a measure of body fat based on your height and weight. The BMI is controversial, and although some people believe it's not accurate enough, I disagree. Although it doesn't give you the underlying fat-to-muscle ratio or take bone structure into account, it is a good tool to guide you when it comes to determining what your healthy weight is. For most people, and most women, it provides an accurate, reasonable, and generous range for healthy weight, and also specifically delineates what is underweight, overweight, and obese. In my opinion, unless you are a bodybuilder, you can trust the BMI chart. You'll find out more about the BMI and I'll give you a chart so you can find out your own number in Chapter 9. In the meantime, no matter what your mother always said, being "big-boned" is no excuse to carry more body fat than is normal for your frame. It's time to stop making excuses!

YOUR VEGETABLE AND FRUIT CONSUMPTION

One of the heart-healthiest ways you can improve your diet is to load it up with vegetables and fruits. Eating well isn't always about what you can't eat, and this is one fantastic exception. It's about what you need to eat *more* of. Isn't that great news?

A lot of people hardly ever eat vegetables, or they eat only one or two different types of vegetables, like lettuce and tomatoes. What a waste! Vegetables are like magic when it comes to vitality. They contain all kinds of nutrients that seem to have a potent effect on health. They deeply nourish you, and they provide you with the real, bioavailable versions of vitamins and minerals that probably have a much more profound (and safer!) effect than that vitamin pill you choke down every morning.

The one diet that has been proven to decrease the incidence of heart disease the most is the Mediterranean diet, which is very high in vegetables and fruits, nuts, grains, olive or canola oil, and everything you would ever want to eat while lying on the beach in Greece. I'll talk much more about diet and the power of produce (plus easy ways to eat more vegetables and fruits) in a later chapter.

YOUR DRINKING

For some reason, when I ask New Yorkers if they drink, they say things like, "No, only one to three glasses of wine with dinner every night." That sounds like drinking to me! Drinking is a way of life for many people, but it's time for you to take your own personal alcohol reality check.

Even though you've probably heard that a little bit of alcohol can actually be good for your heart, excessive alcohol consumption has been linked to an increase in heart disease. Too much alcohol can cause heart palpitations in some people, it can raise blood pressure, and it can damage your liver as well as your heart.

When I recommend a glass of wine a day, what I am telling you is to have a glass of wine with dinner. For women, one glass is recommended, and up to two for men. A single serving is just 4 to 6 ounces of wine or 2 ounces of hard liquor. That's not very much.

I'm not telling you to run right out and start tying one on, because an entire bottle of wine or multiple visits to the keg are much worse than not drinking at all. But if sipping a Bordeaux with your whole-grain pasta and fresh vegetables works for you, then "Cheers!"

YOUR SLEEP

Sleep is nice. It's great when you can get it. But what does it have to do with your heart? Actually, your risk of heart disease goes way up if you get less than six hours of sleep or more than nine hours of sleep per night. In other words, there is a heart-healthy sleep sweet spot, and if you stay within it, you lower your risk.

Sleep is so important for rejuvenation, but we aren't totally sure why too much sleep puts people at risk for heart disease. Is it about being too sedentary? Do those extra hours of sleep translate to fewer hours of exercise? Or is something else involved? Stay tuned for more research on this subject.

We do understand more about how a lack of sufficient sleep causes stress. Sleep helps repair and replenish the sympathetic nervous system. Without that repair, you are likely to suffer from an excess of stress hormones. You'll be more likely to be living on adrenaline, whether from anxiety or too much coffee. So go to bed early tonight! Your heart will thank you.

YOUR STRESS AND LIFE PERCEPTIONS

Stress affects everything. I mean that. Literally everything in your life can be negatively impacted by too much stress. It might just be the most pervasive and significant Heart Throb you can actually control, because managing it smartly will help you to make better decisions about how you really want to live your life. Nothing works well when you are stressed. When you feel calm and in control, everything works better.

We've only recently begun to understand how drastically stress impacts the body, especially in terms of inflammation. High levels of stress hormones can eventually cause inflammation in the body, leading to high blood pressure, obesity, and many of the other Heart Throbs.

In Chapter 11, I will talk more about how you perceive your world, and whether your viewpoint adds to your risk of heart disease, but just knowing that stress, anxiety, and hostility are key players in what happens to your heart is important. Also, how you view the world is critical in how happy your heart is. Whether you see the glass half full or half empty actually makes a big difference in your heart disease risk.

For now, just take a few deep breaths, and maybe go to a yoga class.

These are the Heart Throbs you need to pay attention to in your own life. This is your measuring tape to help you know where you stand. Maybe this is the first time you've realized that your health might not be optimal, and maybe it's time to talk to a nutritionist or a trainer, or enlist your best friend for help. Ask your doctor to do some tests. Take that good hard look in the mirror. You can't take action until you know yourself, and that's what this list is all about.

This isn't just about early diagnosis and early prevention. This is about your choice and how you want to live. Remember, your health is in *your* hands, and you have the total control to live a full, vital, long life. I promise you, you can do it.

Let's start making some changes.

This Chapter, by Heart

♥ If you know your individual Heart Throbs, or signs of wellness or unwellness (as opposed to knowing general population risk factors), you are more likely to take steps to change your life.

♥ A healthy endothelium (the lining of your arteries) is essential for heart health as well as overall health and vitality. Learn what behaviors put the endothelium at risk, and what signs, or Heart Throbs, to look for that suggest your endothelium is already in trouble.

♥ Dr. Steinbaum's Heart Throbs include:

✓ Your Exercise Tolerance
✓ Your Resting Heart Rate
✓ Your Heart Rate Variability
✓ Your Smoking Habit
✓ Your Cholesterol Level
✓ Your Blood Pressure
✓ Your Blood Sugar
✓ Your Inflammation
✓ Your ApoE Genes
✓ Your Hormonal Issues
✓ Your Family History
✓ Your Body Fat
✓ Your Vegetable and Fruit Consumption
✓ Your Drinking
✓ Your Sleep
✓ Your Stress and Life Perceptions

CHAPTER THREE

What You Carry in Your Heart

I have a secret to tell you. If you are one of my patients and we know each other, then please forgive me, because I'm telling your secret. I'm breaking patient confidentiality, but I'm telling my secret too, because honestly, this is no secret. I'm writing it here, in black and white, because of the urgency. Because despite everything we already know about heart disease, this might be the most important thing you learn from this book. Telling this secret is a matter of life and death.

Almost all of my patients confess to me, in hushed, worried, anxious, panicky voices, that they are under stress, and not just stress, but great, unbearable stress—stress far beyond what "normal people" suffer. They are under the most stress. They are the worst possible cases. Their stress is an emergency. It's hurting their hearts. It's killing them. They feel it.

I believe them because I can see it in their eyes.

But what my patients never seem to understand is that they all say this. They are all in the same boat. They all think that they are worst-case scenarios. And they hardly ever admit to anyone else how they feel.

Sometimes my patients are dramatic about their stress. Sometimes they underplay it, as in, "This shouldn't bother me, but . . ." Sometimes they shake their heads and say things like "Nobody knows," or "Nobody gets it," or "Only me." They feel alone.

They all feel alone, and yet they are in the same group, with so much in common. None of them realizes that they all feel the same way, because nobody wants to admit out loud how crushing their stress really is. And many of them, after their confession, finish with the hopeless and helpless statement "Maybe it's all in my head."

I wish I could put all of them in a room together, and all of you reading this book too, so that you could talk to each other and see how you are not alone, how stress is happening to all of us. Many of my younger women patients ask me if they are my youngest patients. I promise them that they are not. My older patients worry that they are going through unusual hormonal issues. They are not. We all feel different, like our problems are unlike anyone else's, but they are not. You are not alone! None of you.

Beyond the Heart Throbs I mentioned in the last chapter—beyond your blood pressure, cholesterol, diet, how much you sit, whether you ate a salad today, beyond all of that—is something that women must understand if they are going to save their own lives: *Stress hurts your heart,* and by association, stress hurts the rest of your body, your mind, and your whole life. That's why you have to do something about it.

In some ways, stress is "in your head" because it starts in your brain, but it quickly spreads everywhere, until you're sweating it out of your pores. Stress can become your life, and that's the fastest way to wither your heart. You can't live a heart-centered life of health and vitality if you are constantly living under the dark heavy slowly sinking ceiling that is stress.

Stress affects you in so many ways that I couldn't possibly explain them all, but one of the most blatant is the way it compromises your ability to make healthy lifestyle choices. Stress keeps you from living for your own benefit. You spend all your time living in the past or the future and missing out on your life. You eat too much and skip exercise because it feels like an immediate remedy, but those things only make stress worse.

I was on the subway the other day and I saw a young mother with a little boy. She was morbidly obese, and her child was quite overweight too. They were both eating potato chips and drinking soda, and she had this look in her eyes, as if all she could think was, "How am I going to get through the day?"

All I could think was, "How is this woman going to make it to age forty?"

Stress can cause you to destroy your health, to go so far past the behaviors you know are good for you that you can't even see your way back again. Or it can keep you from learning what's good for you, if you never really knew. Stress makes you seek out the easy way, the most convenient food, and the least rigorous movement. It makes you avoid the confrontation and step back from what you really want. It can cause anxiety, depression, overeating, or undereating, and it can sap your energy and distract you from your passion. It destroys relationships, jobs, career plans, and health. Simply said, it keeps you from taking good care of yourself, and because of this, it is a killer.

I mean that quite literally. Stress is killing us. Stress is one of the *major contributors* to heart disease. Nobody tells you this when you take on another project or lose your job or get a divorce. Nobody warns you, the way they warn you when you smoke cigarettes or gain too much weight. They don't say, "You'd better not do that or you might take on too much stress!" Instead, we feel judged if we don't do it all, juggle everything, manage every possible aspect of life without help. People with stressed-out, overextended lives are revered in our culture.

Oh, sure, we might make jokes about it. "If I have to do one more thing, make one more call, or answer one more e-mail, I am just going to die!" "If you kids don't stop fighting, you're going to give me a heart attack." "Don't tell me I have to do that too! Are you trying to kill me?" But it's not funny. It's really happening, to men, to women, to *young women.*

If we all knew, really knew, really *accepted* the knowledge that stress hurts our hearts and that it's an epidemic in our culture, maybe we would actually start doing something about it. In this book, I sometimes talk about studies and research results that haven't yet been incorporated into standards of care, but the connection between stress and the heart actually has been proven, time and time again. It's just that doctors won't usually bring it up, because they don't know what to tell you to do about it.

Heart Beats

Stress, anxiety, depression, hostility, and social isolation have all been linked to a higher risk of heart disease. There is a huge connection between the mind and the heart. Chronic stress has been associated with a 2.1-fold increase in the risk of having a heart attack, even after adjusting for age, gender, geographic region, and smoking. The studies prove that mental stress has been associated with heart abnormalities like ischemic ST segments, abnormal myocardial perfusion, decrease in left ventricular ejection fraction, and wall motion abnormalities. That's cardiology-speak, but what it means is that the heart is suffering from oxygen deprivation every time you let your brain steer the course.

Defining Your Stress

What is stress for you? Stress means different things to different people, so no matter how a study might define it, you can only define it for yourself by feeling it. Think about what makes your heart pound or gives you chest pain or that deep central aching. Think about what makes you feel unsettled or uncomfortable or unhappy, like things just aren't in sync. What provokes your emotional response?

Whatever it is, this is where you need to look. Nobody else can do it for you. A doctor can't measure it. A doctor can measure your cholesterol or blood pressure or inflammatory markers, but he can't measure what's going on in your head. And yet the stress you feel is as much of a Heart Throb as high cholesterol or high blood pressure or inflammation. In fact, stress can directly increase inflammation, blood pressure, and cholesterol, but only you can really tell the true effects of your stress.

You can also notice where you carry your stress. Different people tend to carry their stress in different places. Some people get diarrhea. (Yes, I just said diarrhea. It happens to everyone, so relax.) Some people get migraine headaches. Some people can't sleep and some people feel stress directly in their hearts, which can manifest as chest pain, palpitations, shortness of breath, and other heart-related symptoms.

This says something about you. Knowing where you carry your stress is part of knowing who you are, and if you carry stress in your heart, then you are even more vulnerable to developing heart disease. You have to be even more careful. You have to be vigilant and protective—you have to advocate for your own heart, like you would for your own child.

To confuse us further, the physical symptoms of stress or anxiety are remarkably similar to the physical symptoms of a heart attack: increased heart rate, shortness of breath, dizziness, lightheadedness, nausea, abdominal pain, headache, disturbed sleep, fatigue, sleeping too much, sleeping too little, poor concentration, nervousness, irritability, a change in appetite, numbness or tingling of the extremities, sweating, trembling, a feeling of choking, chills, or hot flashes. When I am speaking to a group of people and I list the symptoms of a heart attack, I often see people squirming in their seats. The list of symptoms sounds uncomfortably familiar. Stress and the heart go hand in hand. They mimic each other, until we don't even know what's what. Later in this chapter, I'll show you how to tell the difference between a panic attack and a heart attack, but for now, just consider the significance of the similarities between the effects of what goes on in your mind and a heart attack. They don't mimic each other for nothing. They are intimately related. Each one can trigger the other.

This is why I suggest that your brain be demoted from its status as Chief Operating Officer. It's time to give your heart a chance to run the show. Your brain needs a vacation.

Heart Sense

The most dramatic example of the link between stress and the body is a condition called Takotsubo's cardiomyopathy, or broken heart syndrome. Broken heart syndrome is really the ultimate expression of stress in the body. It occurs when a person is under great stress, or after an emotional shock or trauma. All of the stress hormones surge, increasing the heart rate and blood pressure, and the heart goes into something like a shock state, and stops functioning. It looks just like a heart attack, but the arteries are totally normal. It's a true, pure mind-body connection, but not the kind you ever want to have. The medical community sees it, knows it, and yet we don't know what to do about it to prevent it. It can be fatal. You can literally die of a broken heart.

Women less than 55 years old are nine times more likely to develop this syndrome compared to men, and women older than 55 years old are 2.9 times more at risk. So what does that mean? Are you going to let stress into your life to such an extent that it physically overwhelms your heart? Let's not do that. Let's figure out how to go a different way.

Fight-or-Flight vs. Tend-and-Befriend

I've always been fascinated by the fact that stress damages women's hearts more than it does men's hearts. I wonder why this is. We don't know for sure, but several small studies have demonstrated that stress and anxiety decrease functioning of the arteries of the heart in women. These studies have shown that under stress, women's arteries do not dilate as well as men's. It's your poor endothelium again! Stress can actually damage the endothelium because of the inflammation it triggers in your body. The lining of the arteries becomes stiff and rigid and more easily torn, and that's where the cardiac dysfunction—and life dysfunction—really gets rolling.

But I have a theory about this. Women and men simply deal with stress differently. In stressful situations, men tend to have a fight-or-flight response. They put up their dukes or they run away, physically or emotionally (did I just describe what's been going on in your relationship?). Unfortunately, you can't totally blame him, because it's biological and hormonal. And you can tell him I said that.

You've probably heard about the fight-or-flight response because articles and books about stress talk about it a lot. However, you might have thought this was a universal stress response—in both men and women. Actually, this fight-or-flight response isn't the default response in women. We deal with stress in a different way.

Women are more comfortable feeling the suffering of stress, and helping to fix it in others, rather than running from it or fighting it. We don't like confrontation. We want to *talk about it*. For a long time. In great detail. Until we feel better. (Am I describing your relationship again?)

This response to stress is called tend-and-befriend, and it's practically the opposite of fight-or-flight. Just as fight-or-flight is biologically and hormonally based in men, tend-and-befriend is biologically and hormonally supported in women. Of course, there are many exceptions, but biochemically, men have an antisocial response to stress, and women have a social response to it. That's a major difference— and the cause of a lot of additional stress in relationships!

Women have a tend-and-befriend stress response because of oxytocin, a hormone released in the body during pregnancy, breastfeeding, and lovemaking. This hormone makes us feel calmer, more relaxed, more social, and more loving. If we all lived with more endorphins and oxytocin, the world might be a nicer place.

Oxytocin is both a stress defense, in that it lowers stress hormones in the body, and also a tool for forging social bonds. Oxytocin is reduced by the presence of testosterone, so men have it too, but women have a lot more of it. Because of this, women should be able to handle stress better than men. When the men fight or flee, we can step in and calm everyone down and forge alliances and help get everyone back together. And we do it for ourselves too—we manage our stress by talking, by reaching out to other people, by working it out, verbally and emotionally. We aren't built to handle our stress alone. We're built to handle stress with our social skills, and that village of people around us.

These complementary hormones worked back when someone had

to tend to the home and someone had to go hunt for the food, but now these differing approaches to stress tend to clash.

I'm not trying to be controversial here or offend anybody of either gender. As I said, there are many exceptions—women who fight or flee, and men who tend and befriend. I'm just talking about biochemistry here, and the way it tends to manifest and influence behavior in general.

And here's where I see a big problem for women.

In today's world, tend-and-befriend isn't necessarily part of the schedule. You're super-busy and overextended, and when stress hits you like a sledgehammer, the reality is that you may not have the time for peacemaking or to call a friend or meet with a group to discuss your stress. Maybe you have time to text somebody something to the effect of, "OMG I'm stressed!" but that's not exactly the way tend-and-befriend is meant to defuse your stress. You need face time. Not the iPhone app, but actual face time! You need communication with others. You need to *talk*. But when you can't even find a way to sneak away for a cup of coffee with your BFF, how are you going to have time to befriend your enemy (work rival, jealous family member, unsympathetic teacher)? You may not have time to take care of everyone who is getting hurt by stress in a stressful situation.

You may only have time to fight or flee. It might be all you can manage. So you take on the male version of stress management, and it just *doesn't work very well for you*.

Also, because the fight-or-flight response is so expected, because this is how the media has decided humans in general handle stress, and because in many ways women are still expected to act like men, many women have moved away from their natural impulses and toward a more masculine response to stress. We fight more because that's how to get ahead or get listened to. Or we flee, isolating ourselves and not dealing with the problems in our lives because it's easier than dealing with confrontation and aggression. And that hurts us.

At some point, you might even forget that sitting down and chatting it out with your girlfriends was ever a real option for dealing with stress. And your girlfriends might all be fighting or fleeing too, so they might not even answer the phone, or the text you sent out like a flare, hoping for a rescue. I suspect this displaced stress response is a big part of why we are seeing such an increase in heart disease in younger women.

Women need to have a network, a team, a village. Historically, that was part of the plan, and it wasn't until we really started climbing up that ladder and fighting our way to the top that the posse became less of a priority. Relationships are part of the sustenance of womanhood, both with friends and romantic partners.

I think the tend-and-befriend stress response is also relevant to men in many ways. Studies show that the healthiest people, both male and female, are people who are in happy marriages, who have someone they can turn to and lean on and talk to. However, in couples that are not happy, when there is hostility, an inability to confide in each other, or no positive support, then stress is high in both men and women. People in unhappy relationships experience more worry and anxiety and lower self-esteem, and these emotional effects have been demonstrated to trigger physical changes in the body, which lead to increased sickness and an increase in heart disease.

We all need a team, a support staff, our people, whether it's family, girlfriends, or your partner. You need support. You need to deal with your stress by sharing it, rather than hiding it or fighting it or trying to handle it alone. This is part of what it means to be a woman. And if you are a man, you need this too—you need support. You need someone who you can depend on, even if you don't always want to share every single nuance of your stress. Just knowing someone is there for you eases the burden. Maybe if we managed the stress in small incre-ments, on a daily basis, rather than pushing it aside until the big fire-works happen, we could manage the rush of stress hormones a little better. Maybe therein lies the treatment for broken heart syndrome.

Heart Throbs: A Closer Look

I briefly mentioned the specific psychosocial Heart Throbs in the last chapter, but let's look at them more closely here, because I really want you to recognize yourself in some of the most common ways stress manifests itself. These are Heart Throbs too, and just as real as high blood pressure or cholesterol. So think about these—where do you recognize yourself? And remember, you are not alone. We're all stressed. We've all learned to default to fight-or-flight. And we can find our way back together.

DEPRESSION

Depression is all too common in women. One in four women will experience severe depression at some point in her life, and depression affects twice as many women as men, regardless of other factors like racial and ethnic background or income. Only about 20 percent of depressed women ever seek treatment, and despite what I said about how happily married people are healthier, married women are more likely to experience depression than single women. At highest risk are young mothers who stay at home with their small children. We think that having young children should be a time of bliss, but for some of us, this period is isolating, challenging, lonely, and difficult. Many people have been on antidepressants at some point or another, even though most people don't like to advertise the fact.

Depression isn't a benign condition. It damages relationships, it destroys lives, and it hurts your heart. Depression may seem like something that is "in your head," but it's a major Heart Throb, especially for perimenopausal and menopausal women. If you have any sign of depression while going into menopause, it's very important to address it, not just to yourself but by telling your doctor. Depression often goes hand in hand with heart disease.

Depression puts you at risk for heart disease because it actually changes the hormone balance, increases sympathetic tone, and raises your heart rate and blood pressure. It contracts the arteries, increases the release of stress hormones like cortisol, which leads to inflammation, and increases platelet activation, which leads to sticky platelets that can cause heart attacks.

Depression's ill effects aren't just about your biochemistry. People who are depressed tend to isolate themselves and are less likely to seek out social support. They also smoke more and drink more alcohol and make poor dietary choices, eating too many starchy and sugary foods or just eating too much. They don't exercise as much. They get tired. They don't feel like taking their medications.

Sometimes depression happens before heart disease strikes, and it is very common after a heart attack or bypass surgery for women and men of any age. Women generally recover worse than men after a heart attack, especially if they are diagnosed with depression, and younger women are even more likely to be depressed and have worse outcomes than men after heart events.

Knowing whether depression is a problem for you is the first step in addressing it. There are several depression scales doctors use to diagnose clinical depression, but the simplest one I've ever seen asks just two questions. It's not going to diagnose you in any complex way, but it can tell you whether you might have a problem and whether you should seek some help.

Just answer these two questions honestly:

1. During the past two weeks, have you often been bothered by feeling down, depressed, or hopeless?

2. During the past two weeks, have you often been bothered by feeling little interest or pleasure in doing things you normally enjoy?

If you answered yes to either one of these questions, then you might be clinically depressed. If you answered yes to both questions, your chances are even higher. (If you answered no to both of them but started crying while reading them, then you are just not being honest with yourself.)

This is the time to tell yourself the absolute truth. There is evidence that people who find out they have an illness or who experience an upsetting event and choose to ignore it or forget about it (this is called repressive behavior) actually experience physical symptoms of elevated stress, like a measurable increase in stress hormones, with every denial response.

That means every time you say, "I'm fine" when you aren't, you are pumping yourself full of inflammation-causing stress hormones. Not addressing the issue isn't the way to handle it, even if it's the way most people tend to handle their most intense feelings.

So let's address the issue. Let's tend and befriend. So what if the medical community doesn't know how to help you? Maybe we can find a way to help you help yourself.

No matter what any study might say about which treatments for depression do or don't work, you need to find what will work for you. Maybe it will be an antidepressant. They have helped millions, billions—who knows? Maybe therapy or counseling would completely change your life. Or maybe the answer is simpler. Maybe getting a good night's sleep is all you need. Maybe you just need an extra set of hands or a shoulder to cry on and you'll start to feel better. Maybe you just need to admit to someone, out loud, how miserable you feel—someone who will listen without judgment.

Or maybe you need some time to go exercise, or meet with your friends, or take a bath alone, with nobody asking you for anything. Maybe you need just one morning per week when someone else gets up with the baby and you can actually sleep in. Only you know what you need, but first you have to admit the need to yourself. Maybe you just need to admit you might need a little help. It's not the end of the world. We all need help sometimes. Let someone tend and befriend *you*.

And if you do seek out therapy, action-oriented counseling is the best, especially for people who are working with a medical issue. You might not need someone to help you dig deep into your childhood traumas. What you really need is someone who can help you start to feel better now. You need to get the help to reframe this situation you are in. It's never easy to feel un-well, physically or emotionally, or even to feel not like yourself. Sometimes just getting a new perspective makes all the difference in the world. Find someone who can help you make an action plan you can start working on right now. Someone who can help foster the optimism you may have lost, the positive attitude you need to reacquire, the hope for your future you can reclaim, and the self-love you may have left on the curb.

A lot of people have been in therapy, even if they haven't admitted it. If we all speak up about our experiences, we would all feel so much better. We would know we aren't alone. So ask trusted friends: Who do they recommend? Do they know a good therapist? Try your local hospital and see if there are some recommendations there. Then shop around. If you don't like someone, don't go back. Keep looking. You have the right to find someone who can really help you, someone you connect with, someone who can point you in the right direction. We all comparison shop for lots of things. The least you can do is find a high-quality guide when you are readjusting your thoughts.

And even if you don't go the therapy route, make a change. Talk it out. Forge those social connections. Don't be afraid. This is your life we're talking about here. This is your heart. Let someone help you make a plan for how you can start feeling better. Once this action plan is your own, then it is all yours, and once it is all yours, then you can act on it and begin to make changes and look at the world in a slightly different way. Little by little, step by step, and thought by thought, you make small adjustments. Before you know it, things start to look up.

ANXIETY

Although many stress symptoms can mimic a heart attack, an anxiety attack can be a dead ringer. When someone has an anxiety or panic attack, these are the symptoms:

- Shortness of breath
- Rapid heart rate
- Rapid breathing
- Chest pain
- Sweating
- Numbness and tingling
- Nausea
- Dizziness

These are the same symptoms of a heart attack, so how do you know you're not having a heart attack when this happens?

Sometimes you don't. Sometimes patients come in to the hospital thinking they are having a heart attack and it turns out to be an anxiety or panic attack. In fact, this has kept many women from seeking treatment for a heart attack. They were afraid it was only in their heads. They were afraid of looking silly. They were afraid of being admitted for a heart attack, only to find out they didn't have one. To have the doctors shake their heads in annoyance, the nurses whisper and roll their eyes, "Oh, it was only a panic attack."

But this is just the attitude that makes anxiety worse, and it's a completely unfounded distinction. An anxiety attack is *not* just "in your head." It has real, measurable, physical effects in your body, including your heart, where it can be associated with a racing heart, shortness of breath, dizziness and feelings of passing out, and chest pain. It ends up in your heart, even if it doesn't start there. If you are sitting in a cardiologist's office with symptoms in your heart, it's your body, and it's all connected.

But you don't have to be a victim to a panic attack. We know that when somebody has an anxiety attack, they often experience shortness of breath about forty-five minutes before the panic attack happens. You might not notice it, but the effect of this shortness of breath is a change in the acid-base balance in the body, because that is affected by the way you breathe. This is how the numbness and tingling begin. The rest of the anxiety attack is like a snowball rolling downhill. It starts with the breath, and it gets bigger and bigger. But because an anxiety attack starts with breathing too quickly, you can also stop it by slowing down your breath.

Here's a little trick I give my anxiety-prone patients: When you breathe deeply, you send a message to your body that everything is okay. It stimulates the parasympathetic nervous system associated with calmness and resting. Shallow fast breathing, on the other hand, signals an emergency, sending your body into high-stress mode. So at the first sign of a panic attack or feelings of anxiety, take in a deep breath to the slow count of four, in through the nose. Hold it for four counts, then let it out vigorously with a loud *shhh* sound for six counts. After you've exhaled, hold for another four counts. Repeat this a few times.

Once you turn on that parasympathetic nervous system, it takes over, decreases your heart rate, decreases your blood pressure, decreases your respiratory rate, and forces your body back to normal. It is a quick fix when you feel that anxiety creeping up on you. This won't work for a heart attack, so if your symptoms begin to slow down and disappear after you do this, then you've just taken control of your own anxiety, and saved your heart from the experience too. Score one for you—you are back in control.

If it doesn't change anything, then call your doctor or go to the emergency room. Even if they determine you didn't have a heart attack, it's better to be safe and sure. Never be afraid to seek medical help if you think you might be having a heart attack! Too many women make that mistake. They think it's only in their heads when it's really, truly, fatally in their hearts.

Besides, just because you aren't having a heart attack at the moment you feel chest pain, nausea, and dizziness doesn't mean the event is irrelevant to your heart. It has everything to do with your heart, your future, and how symptoms of stress play out in your individual, completely unique body. It might not be a heart attack this time, but next time? You, of all people, need to take care of your heart, because your heart is holding the burden of your stress.

If anxiety is the way you express your stress, think about where it comes from. In my experience, a lot of anxiety is based on fantasy, not reality. Are you telling yourself a story that isn't true? Are you making up something that hasn't happened? Do you obsess about what's going to happen to you in the future or what could potentially happen to someone you love? This is a habit, just like negative thinking. You have the power to stop yourself when you recognize your pattern and remind yourself that the source of your worry isn't real.

Inhale. Hold. Exhale. Hold. Then ask yourself what you really know to be true. This is all part of shifting your attitude and flipping the switch on the stress response. You can look at any situation in any number of ways. Try a different way, a new story, if the one you're using isn't working for you. (And if it's causing anxiety, then it's definitely not working for you.)

Sometimes active relaxation practices can also help calm obsessive or anxious thoughts. Listen to calming music and focus on the sound rather than on your worries. Breathe deeply and slowly, to let your body know everything is all right. Talk to someone—a friend, a therapist or counselor, a family member, or anyone who can help you put your worries into perspective. Remember, tend and befriend. Find someone who will make you feel better, not worse, even if it's just for a five-minute conversation, to let it all out. Sometimes voicing your anxieties out loud deflates them completely, and you realize, without anyone even telling you, how unfounded your fears really were.

PESSIMISM

Recently, multiple studies have linked pessimism with poor health and poor healing after a health problem. It is fascinating that the way you choose to see the world could be so dramatically influential in how your body chooses to maintain or regain its health and balance.

I believe pessimism is linked to both depression and anxiety. If you tend to default to the negative viewpoint, if you find yourself thinking and saying the word "no" a lot, if you have that pervasive feeling that things really aren't going to work out for you, then you are setting your heart up for failure. I mean this literally. In patients who already had a heart attack, those with a pessimistic attitude had a 30 percent higher death rate than optimists, even when the study controlled for other factors. The pessimism alone increased the death rate.

Some people believe that pessimism is a personality trait, but I believe it's a habit. You learn it, or maybe you default to it naturally, but that doesn't mean you can't start nudging yourself in the other direction. Optimism is one of the most potent healers and preventive measures a person can take for a long, healthy life, and it's completely within your reach. Optimism makes life so much more enjoyable. Nothing is more precious than when you can wake up every morning and say that life is good and you are going to have the best day you possibly can.

I used to say to my son every morning while opening the shades to wake him up, "Good morning, Sun, and welcome to a brand-new day." One morning, when it was raining, I came into his room to wake him up, opened the shades, and said, "Oops! I can't welcome the sun today."

"Mommy, even when the sun doesn't come out, it's still a brand-new day," he said, in his matter-of-fact way. That made my day. He learned optimism from me—and then he taught it to me!

ANGER AND HOSTILITY

Anger and hostility aren't traits traditionally associated with women, but oh my goodness, the anger and hostility I've seen in my office defy all the stereotypes! Women are angry, men are angry, and it causes some of the most dramatic stress responses in the body of all the emotions. Holding anger and hostility in your heart is so toxic, and taking it out on other people is even worse. Study after study has linked anger and hostility with heart disease. In one large trial called the WISE (Women's Ischemia Syndrome Evaluation) trial, some of the women who had severe chest pain they thought was due to heart disease, but who didn't have any artery blockages that showed up on an angiogram, turned out to have major issues with anger and hostility. It is possible that the emotions alone were causing physical chest pain.

Is this you? Are you angry? Are you hostile? Do you keep pushing it down into your heart so you don't have to experience it? If this sounds familiar, then you've got to change something, my friend, or you will hurt your heart sooner or later. Getting along with others is so important for emotional well-being. We are social creatures, like it or not. I've seen the research that shows that those who get along better with their neighbors, relatives, and friends are less likely to have health problems. We know this intuitively. It makes sense. We know it feels healthy to be supportive of others and to let others support us. But when something's triggered your anger, it can be hard to get back to that place.

There is an art to releasing hostility. The people who take their hostility and put it on a silver platter and deliver it to their family and friends and partners every day actually do worse, health-wise, than the people who repress it, but the repressors do much worse than the people who are able to let it go.

If you need help managing your anger, please, please seek out someone who is professionally able to give you the tools to do this. Go find a punching bag, start running, get on the floor and do as many push-ups as you need to until it is gone, leave the room, go outside and walk around the block. Disperse it, dispel it, and let it go.

Or hash it out with someone who isn't the subject of your anger, until you've gotten back to the place where you can tend and befriend again.

We'll keep talking about this throughout the book. We'll work it out, but just start by giving it some thought. What are you really angry about? You don't have to answer it yet. Just ask yourself.

JOB DISSATISFACTION

Women in the workforce who are unhappy with their jobs are at a higher risk of heart disease, according to some recent studies that specifically pinpointed the feeling of not having control over their day as the source of the stress that triggers the risk. The women who felt the most stress were not those in high-pressure supervisory positions, even though we might expect that. Isn't the boss the one under all the pressure? Actually, the truly stressed employees were in staff or service positions or other positions where they were not in charge.

Of course, you can't always change your job, so the key here, when you are not technically in charge of your day, is to be in charge of your perception of your day, your job, your position, and your self-worth.

YOUR OUTLOOK

So much of stress comes down to outlook. Babies are attracted to happy, smiling faces, but studies have demonstrated that as we age, we become more likely to gravitate toward sad or miserable faces. We tend to be more drawn to the negative. Why is it that as we get older, the glass becomes half empty? Being drawn to things and people that are happy and engaging and optimistic might be all you need to change your perspective. We don't always have control over what is happening in our lives, but we can be proactive about our perspective. I'll talk a lot in this book about how to reframe your perspective to one that's more heart-centered. I know how bleak everything could look, but if you can stop telling yourself stories, you just might be able to see all the wonderful, heart-healing possibilities in your future.

This Chapter, by Heart

♥ Chronic stress is one of the biggest heart disease risks for women.

♥ Common ways stress manifests in women are as depression, anxiety, pessimism, anger, hostility, job dissatisfaction, and outlook.

♥ You can learn the art of reframing situations and reorienting your perspective to help reduce stress in your life and lower your risk for heart disease.

CHAPTER FOUR

The Heart of the Matter

If you can actually, physically see something, you're more likely to think about it. You're more likely to prioritize it, and it's more likely to feel real to you. Look down for a minute. See your breasts? There they are, right down there next to your sternum (more or less). You see them when you get dressed in the morning, when you get undressed at night, and when you wear something that makes them look particularly . . . noticeable. (You know which dress I mean.) So when something goes wrong with your breasts—you feel a mass, for example—that means something to you. You know something is wrong. You get it checked out. You can wrap your head around the fact that breast cancer is a real risk to your health, because there they are, the girls in all their glory, and you'd rather they stayed healthy, thank you very much.

But the heart? There it is, right behind your breasts, unglamorously doing its job all day long without fanfare, without bothering anyone. You can't see it, you can't hear it, you can't usually feel it, and you definitely can't touch it, so it might not seem quite as real to you as your breasts, or your face, or your arms and legs, or your hair, or anything else you can see in the mirror. It's obvious to you when you're having a bad-hair day, but how will you know if you're having a bad-heart day?

Now that you understand the areas where your heart might be at risk, I want you to understand your heart itself—what it looks like, how it works, and what is actually going on when something isn't working correctly. Because you can't see it, hear it, or touch it, it may seem like your heart isn't really worth thinking about—that is, until something happens to it. Until it skips a beat, or goes too fast, or doesn't catch up to you when you are playing ball, or worse of course, until it stops. It could be hurt or feel pressure or it might not be working right and you might feel nothing at all, but you need to know what's going on in there. When you understand your heart, you'll be less alarmed at minor symptoms, but you'll also be more inclined to do what's right and best for your most important internal organ.

I believe what happens when women can't see their hearts is that they either blow their worries all out of proportion because they don't really know how the heart works or they totally ignore heart health because the heart is out of sight and out of mind. I think if we could see it, touch it, and really know what it is doing, we might respect it more, help it along, and have a more realistic view of its role in our lives.

This is my goal in this chapter. You need to know what that invisible metronome and pumper of life is doing in there, and how it is working. That way you can learn not only to appreciate but to actually visualize your heart. And maybe then you'll be even more motivated to keep it functioning at its very best.

Your Hypochondriac Heart

Years ago, I traveled to the Caribbean with a group of girlfriends because one of them was getting married. We were all staying in a hotel together, and one evening there was a power outage. All the lights went off, and we were all quiet for a moment, and then one of the girls started screaming, "I'm blind! Help me! I'm blind!"

This is what we tend to do. We have a symptom, and if it's a heart-related symptom, and we can't see our hearts and we don't really understand how they work, we freak out. We assume the worst when what's really going on might be some minor glitch in the electrical system.

Things can go wrong with our hearts, and they often do. We know this. But understanding what's going on in your heart will make the whole process a lot less terrifying. The thing I find so interesting about the heart is that it's so metaphorical. It's not just a physical organ that pumps blood. It's the emotional center of your life, and it's literally affected by so much that you do. The heart is affected by hormones as well as emotions, stress as well as love, joy and happiness and laughter and emotional pain and hurt and despair.

I believe it is crucial to address both the metaphorical and physical aspects of the heart because they are so intimately connected. What the mind believes about the heart, what you feel about your heart, and the physical state of your heart are woven together so that each part affects the other. This is why I want you to feel like you know your heart as well as you know your thighs or breasts or hair or your own face. When you understand what's physically true about the heart, it can ease your worry and increase your confidence, which helps us better negotiate the metaphorical side of heart health. This will be painless, I promise—this is an "Everything I Know About the Heart I Learned in Kindergarten" approach. I've explained this to my son, Spencer, who happens to be in kindergarten, and he understands it, so I know you will too.

How the Heart Is Built

There are four parts to the heart:

- The arteries, which carry oxygen-filled blood to all the cells of the body

- The muscles, which beat the blood out of the heart and relax when the heart fills with blood

- The electrical system, which regulates the beating of the heart

- The valves, which control the flow of blood in the right direction between the heart chambers and the body

The heart is divided into a right side and a left side, and inside the heart are four chambers, like four different rooms. The top two rooms are the right atrium and the left atrium. The bottom two rooms are the right ventricle and the left ventricle.

The left side of the heart contains blood filled with oxygen. The heart's job, simply put, is to pump this oxygen to every part of the body. Every cell in your body needs oxygen to function. The heart delivers this oxygen-rich blood through the aorta, which is the largest artery in your whole body. The aorta originates from the left ventricle and extends all the way down to your abdomen. Its branches feed blood to every cell in the body, from the brain to the tips of the toes. Once that oxygen-rich blood gets to the organs and the cells take the oxygen out of the blood, the blood doesn't have oxygen anymore, so it has to go get more.

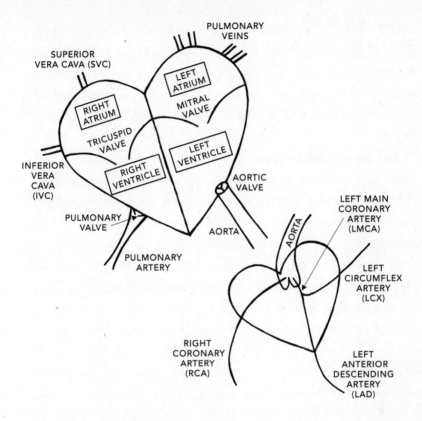

This is the heart diagram I draw for all of my patients to show them how the heart is built.

Now the right side of your heart gets involved. This is the de-oxygenated side of your heart. The blood, now devoid of oxygen, gets pumped back up into the right side of the heart through two primary veins, called the superior vena cava and the inferior vena cava. These veins deliver the deoxygenated blood into the right atrium of your heart. Remember that your heart has no oxygen on the right side. After it goes into the right atrium and then down into the right ventricle, it's delivered through the pulmonary vessels to the lungs to pick up the oxygen that enters our bodies when we breathe.

How incredibly cool is that? The simple act of breathing ultimately takes care of the heart by infusing the blood with vital oxygen again so it can keep the body going. Once the blood gets freshly oxygenated, it gets pumped back to the left side of the heart, and the whole process starts all over again. The arteries always handle the oxygenated blood, and the veins always handle the deoxygenated blood.

In between the four chambers are valves. Think of them as the doors to the four rooms. The aortic valve is the main one that goes through the body from the heart, delivering oxygenated blood to all your major organs, including your heart. It has three cusps, or doors, so when it is closed, it looks like a Mercedes-Benz sign. It is usually really easy to see and to tell if one of those valves is too tight and needs to be fixed (this could happen from an abnormality from birth called a bicuspid aortic valve, from hypertension, or due to aging).

The pulmonary valve, which leads to the lungs, lets blood into the lungs. In between the rooms on the top of the heart and the rooms on the bottom of the heart there are also valves. The valve on the right is the tricuspid valve, which has three leaflets. On the left side, there's the mitral valve, which looks something like French doors with its two leaflets, although it has a lot of different parts to it holding it in place.

While the aorta delivers all this oxygen to your vital organs, it also delivers it to all of the heart's muscles because they need oxygen to function too. The aorta branches off into the left main coronary artery, leading to two other main arteries: the left anterior descending artery down the front of the heart and the left circumflex artery around the side of it. The aorta also branches out around the right side and under the heart to include the right coronary artery.

The left anterior descending artery, left circumflex artery, and right coronary artery branch out as well. It is this network that delivers oxygen to the heart so it can pump. If any of these arteries get narrowed by plaque or blocked completely by a plaque rupture (when a piece breaks off and blocks the passageway), your heart won't get oxygen, and that's what causes a heart attack.

Glitches in the Machine

As you can see, the heart has an amazingly simple yet ingenious design that keeps your entire body nourished and alive. But sometimes things go wrong, often related to your own decisions about your lifestyle. Let's look at some of the things that can go wrong when you don't live from and for the heart.

YOUR ARTERIES

Remember the endothelium, that arterial lining that I compared to the lining of your purse in Chapter 2? When cholesterol, inflammatory cells, smooth muscle cells, macrophages, collagen, and other invaders slip through the little cuts in the lining of your arteries caused by inflammation, smoking, a poor diet, lack of exercise, and the other Heart Throbs I told you about in Chapter 2, the arterial wall can build up plaque. Now, the truth is that plaque can stay there forever and never cause a problem if it is stable and managed with the best diet, exercise, and sometimes medication. However, the plaque can build up so much that it actually impedes the blood flow in the artery. Or, the plaque can rupture and break apart.

When this happens, platelets—the component of blood responsible for clotting—come to seal off the damage, like National Guard troops responding to a disaster. The problem is that the dimensions of the arteries are a bit small for all these troops, so, as the platelets seal off the plaque rupture, the flow of blood down the artery can get blocked and oxygen cannot be delivered effectively. When the delivery of oxygen is impeded, this is called *ischemia.* When it is blocked off completely, you have a heart attack, because supplying oxygenated blood to itself is one of the heart's important jobs. If the blood can't get through, the heart can't function. Most plaque ruptures happen in arteries that are only 30 to 50 percent blocked, a level of blockage that doesn't even show up on a stress test. Ruptures come from those plaques that are unstable and filled with cholesterol, oxidized LDL, and inflammatory cells waiting to burst open with the slightest irritation, like smoking or high blood pressure.

Women tend to have another problem with the arteries: diffuse disease, and a dispersed buildup of plaque rather than a discrete blockage that's easy to spot. A slow buildup of plaque can reduce oxygen delivery in multiple areas at once. This can cause heart symptoms that can be difficult for a doctor to diagnose because no one area is obviously in trouble.

Similarly, women often get subtle plaque erosions rather than one large chunk of plaque breaking off or rupturing. This slow plaque erosion causes multiple minor injuries to the heart. When this happens, a woman may get chest pain, but not severe enough for her to go to the hospital. These are what we used to call "silent heart attacks," which are referred to as *acute coronary syndromes.* These result in little areas of damage to the cells of the heart, instead of the full wall thickness damage of a massive heart attack. Often, when a woman has an undiagnosed or even unsuspected acute coronary syndrome, a doctor will later be able to see the damage in the heart, and the woman may say she doesn't even remember feeling any chest pain. (This can happen to men too, but it occurs more often in women.)

What's scary is that you can have a heart attack when your arteries are just 50 percent blocked, and our traditional testing doesn't detect these blockages. In fact, 68 percent of the time, the blockages that cause a heart attack are less than 50 percent. Only 14 percent of heart attacks reveal blockages of 70 percent or greater, which is the lowest level that a stress test can detect. If that's not a reason to get any and all plaque under control by changing your lifestyle, I don't know what is.

Another thing that can happen with arteries is that they can spasm. A spasm in the coronary artery can suddenly narrow the artery, slowing or completely blocking blood flow to the heart. This can happen due to plaque buildup, but it can also happen in a plaque-free artery. It can be triggered by extreme stress, as well as certain medications or drugs, including cocaine and even tobacco, and possibly by some of the psychological issues that we already discussed.

Heart Beats

In a major trial on women and heart disease called the WISE (Women's Ischemia Syndrome Evaluation) trial, about 50 percent of the women who were referred for angiograms (an invasive test that shows blockages in the arteries) because of chest pain showed no blockages. This was unexpected, because chest discomfort is usually associated with a 70 percent blockage or greater, yet these women appeared to be "fine." But many of them did end up developing heart disease. We don't fully understand why, but I suspect the reason is that these women were experiencing these subtle plaque erosions or arterial spasms. We wouldn't have been able to see either of these on the angiogram, but we now have techniques to help us detect these issues, called IVUS, or Intervascular Ultrasound. This is one of the top ten questions about women and heart disease I told you about in the beginning of this book. We are still seeking the answers. Why did these women have chest pain, and why did they go on to develop heart disease when we couldn't see it? This is just one more reason why heart disease can be such a mystery in women.

Arterial problems are not just heart problems. As I've mentioned before, your arteries go through your entire body, from brain to feet. When there is disease to the arteries to the brain, it is called carotid artery disease. When there is disease to the arteries of the heart, it is called coronary artery disease. When there is disease to the arteries of the legs, it is called peripheral arterial disease (PAD). There are arteries to the kidneys, arteries in the brain, and arteries in the eye. There are arteries throughout the body that become diseased and lead to sickness. Vascular disease often occurs throughout the arteries in the body, so when one area is diseased, it is not uncommon for another part of the body to have a problem as well. The disease is a problem of the endothelium, and that lining is inside every single artery throughout the body. When we live from the heart, we protect our entire bodies.

Heart Beats

In one study of patients who had a stroke, which would be a problem of the carotid arteries leading to the brain, 60 percent had coronary artery disease and 30 percent had peripheral arterial disease (PAD). In those patients who had PAD, 70 percent had coronary artery disease and 40 percent had carotid artery disease. Among those who had coronary artery disease, 30 percent had carotid disease and 26 percent had PAD. In other words, when you have disease in your arteries, it often affects multiple arterial systems. When you practice prevention for the heart, you are protecting all the arteries in your body and decreasing your chances not just of developing coronary artery disease but of developing all kinds of arterial dysfunction.

The bottom line here is that problems in the arteries are usually the result of a lack of blood flow to the muscle of the heart, causing damage. Diagnoses of arterial problems might include:

- Atherosclerosis, which is a buildup of plaque in the arteries

- Acute coronary syndrome, which describes minor damage to the heart muscle, often due to a plaque rupture or erosions

- Heart attack, also called myocardial infarction, which describes major damage to the heart muscle for a variety of arterial-related reasons, such as plaque rupture, arterial blockage, arterial spasm, or even dissection or tearing of an artery

Fortunately, arterial care is surprisingly easy. It's all about taking care of those Heart Throbs from Chapter 2. When you manage the lifestyle factors that contribute to plaque formation, then you reduce plaque, not just in the heart but also in the brain, the carotid artery, the legs—everywhere.

YOUR HEART MUSCLE

Heart muscle function is one of the most crucial aspects of heart health. The muscle is the part that actually beats. When the muscle is strong, your heart beats in a strong, steady, regular rhythm, pushing or pumping the blood through the body, back to the lungs, and back to the heart. In a healthy, undamaged heart, a measure of heart muscle function, called the ejection fraction (the amount of blood pumped out of the ventricle with each heartbeat), is about 55 to 70 percent.

The real reason it's important to prevent plaque in the coronary arteries is because arterial blockages cause damage to the heart muscle, and heart muscle damage is what makes people very ill. When the heart muscle gets damaged, then the ejection fraction goes down. When it goes down far enough, it indicates that the muscle is so weak, it can't pump out the blood the body needs. We call this heart failure. Heart failure means the heart is not pumping enough blood through the body, and it can happen because of a heart attack or for many other reasons. It is often considered the end-stage result of atherosclerosis (blockages in the arteries).

Other things can go wrong with the heart muscle. Inflammation of the lining that surrounds the heart, or the pericardium, is called pericarditis. Chest pain that changes with different positions is a classic symptom of pericarditis. Sometimes inflammation affects the heart muscle itself, which is called myocarditis.

Another common problem with the heart muscle is diastolic dysfunction, which can be associated with a high diastolic blood pressure number (the bottom number in a blood pressure reading). Diastolic dysfunction causes the heart muscle to stiffen, which can cause a form of heart failure called restrictive cardiomyopathy, characterized by the inability of the heart muscle to relax between beats. This is the cause of heart failure that often occurs in women with a long history of high blood pressure. Prevention often involves blood pressure control (through lifestyle or medication) and maintaining a regular exercise regimen. Diastolic dysfunction can become a debilitating disease if it is not treated.

YOUR HEART'S ELECTRICAL SYSTEM

Your heart muscle contracts with each heartbeat, and your electrical system tells your heart when to actually beat. There is an automatic switch for the top part of the heart (the atrium) and there is a switch for the bottom part of the heart (the ventricles). These switches are connected, like a string of lights that extends from the top of the atrium, along the ventricle, down through the middle of the heart, and back up along the sides. I remember once when I was in Kansas City, Missouri, at a lighting ceremony during the holidays, and there was a string of lights all around the city. First one went on, and then all of a sudden, they all turned on one after another with a *ch ch ch ch* sound. That's how I think of the heart's electrical system.

These switches are automatically triggered by the body's "battery," or the autonomic nervous system. This is why you never have to think about turning your heart on or off, or regulating how fast it beats, because it is all automatic. If your body needs your heart to beat faster or slower, the autonomic nervous system takes care of that.

However, sometimes there are glitches in the system, like when one of the Christmas lights goes out or they begin flashing in an irregular rhythm. When you have irregular beats, called arrhythmias, this is an electrical system issue. Early beats in the top or bottom parts of the heart can be caused by dehydration, stress, alcohol, caffeine, electrolyte abnormalities, or stimulants like diet pills, decongestants, or some ADD meds, as well as drugs like cocaine. Obviously, quitting substances that cause these is a good idea. Extra beats coming from the ventricle (the bottom part of the heart) sometimes can be well managed with magnesium supplements such as magnesium glycinate, which is one of the most absorbable forms of magnesium. If the irregular beats cause symptoms, like bothersome palpitations or fluttering in the chest or shortness of breath, medication may be required. If they happen multiple times in a row or there has been any damage to the heart muscle, that warrants further investigation. Sometimes these beats are a sign of blockages in the arteries or of damage to the heart muscle, and in these situations, they could be dangerous.

There are different kinds of irregular beats, named for the area, or "room," of the heart where they occur. Extra early beats on the bottom of the heart are called premature ventricular contractions. These aren't dangerous if they happen one at a time and the heart function is normal. Atrial premature contractions are also common. Sometimes these happen in short "runs," like a series of beats. These are more annoying than dangerous, although if you have other health problems, they could become dangerous and have been associated with strokes, so they are worth telling your doctor about. These extra beats can come from dehydration, stress, caffeine, alcohol, and lack of sleep.

The most common arrhythmia I see in younger women that needs some type of intervention through medication or a procedure is a supraventricular tachycardia, which is an abnormal beat coming from the top part of the heart associated with palpitations (pounding and pitter-patter of the heart), dizziness, and fainting. If you have pounding in your chest, palpitations, butterflies, or the feeling of choking on your heartbeat, chances are you probably have a premature beat somewhere, and it is worth getting it checked out.

Atrial fibrillation is a form of an irregular heartbeat where the atrium doesn't exactly beat. It just fibrillates (individual muscle fibers twitching in a disorganized way), so the pumping isn't effective. Common symptoms of atrial fibrillation include palpitations, fatigue, poor exercise tolerance, shortness of breath, chest pain, feeling of passing out, fainting, edema (fluid that develops in the ankles), and generalized weakness. In people over age 65, atrial fibrillation is occurring in epidemic proportions. About 2.5 million Americans, or about 1 percent of the population, have this condition. Atrial fibrillation often occurs in conjunction with hypertension (high blood pressure), or if the left atrium dilates.

Atrial fibrillation is also associated with alcohol consumption, and people can go into atrial fibrillation after binge drinking. This has been termed "holiday heart syndrome." Alcohol is toxic to the heart muscle and can lead to electrical system irregularity when consumed too often.

The treatment of atrial fibrillation is dependent on the length of time the atrial fibrillation exists and the heart's function. Paroxysmal atrial fibrillation occurs intermittently, and stops on its own. Persistent atrial fibrillation lasts for more than seven days, but it stops with treatment. Permanent atrial fibrillation won't respond to treatment. Your doctor can diagnose which type of atrial fibrillation you have through the use of a heart monitor. (I'll talk more about heart monitors in Chapter 8.)

One of the greatest concerns with atrial fibrillation is the development of strokes, because when blood isn't flowing through the body correctly and collects and pools in the heart, it can clot and the clots can be thrown into the brain. ("Throwing a clot" is medical lingo meaning that a clot breaks loose and travels somewhere in the body where it shouldn't go, like the heart or the brain.) Some people have atrial fibrillation and don't have any structural disease or heart disease or lung disease, and these people are at low risk for throwing a clot that could cause a stroke. Those who are at greatest risk for having a stroke are over the age of 75, have had a previous stroke or TIA (a mini stroke), heart failure, high blood pressure, or diabetes. Their bodies aren't functioning as efficiently, and they tend to have underlying arterial issues, so the clot may break loose and cause trouble. Women with atrial fibrillation are more likely than men to suffer a stroke.

Atrial fibrillation doesn't necessarily kill you, although the incidence of death has been shown to be higher in those who have it. However, sometimes people have significant symptoms of fatigue, palpitations, or shortness of breath, and this may be debilitating or impair the quality of life. By 2050, the prevalence of atrial fibrillation is expected to more than double because atrial fibrillation is often the end result of high blood pressure or valve disease, both of which are associated with the aging population. If we don't pay attention to our hearts, atrial fibrillation can sneak up on us.

Other heart rhythm issues include a too-slow heartbeat, called bradycardia, which can cause cardiac syncope (fainting or a loss of consciousness due to a slow heart rhythm that doesn't push enough blood to your brain), and tachycardia, which is an increased heart rate. Tachycardia can be due simply to a fast heart rate (such as you might have if you are out of shape), or it can be a symptom of another problem.

The most dangerous rhythm to occur that is abnormal is a ventricular tachycardia, which can cause sudden death. Don't panic—this usually occurs in rare situations or when doctors already know your heart isn't functioning well or if there are blockages in the arteries.

Arrhythmias aren't the only electrical issues. Damage or dysfunction in the heart muscle can also cause a delay in the heart's electrical current. This is called a bundle branch block, or heart block. When there are multiple blocks or delays in the electric system, it can lead to fainting. When the "string of lights" doesn't work correctly, from the automatic switch on top to the switch in the ventricles, the transmission of those impulses to prompt a heartbeat are delayed, which can cause you to faint. A pacemaker can regulate the transmission and keeps your heart beating regularly.

YOUR HEART VALVES

Last of all, let's talk about your heart valves. The valves are the passageways or doors between the rooms in your heart, or between your heart and the rest of your body, and if they close tightly, all is well. Chambers of the heart fill with blood, then the valves open to let the blood into the next chamber, then close again. The "bump bump" that you hear and that you call your "heartbeat" is the closing of the valves. The amount of pressure and the amount of volume that the heart has in each one of the chambers depends on when the doors open and close, so the valves need to open correctly, close tightly, and operate in sync.

The heart valves prevent the backflow of blood into your heart, and they also help the heart fill with blood efficiently, get rid of blood effectively, and move blood from room to room or from the heart to other organs. However, if the valves are loose or leaking because they don't close tightly enough or because a genetic abnormality keeps them from closing, or if they are too tight and can't open correctly, then the blood can regurgitate or not flow sufficiently or even flow backward through the heart. This can cause shortness of breath, palpitations, swelling of the ankles, or a particular kind of cough.

Sometimes valve disease requires surgery, but sometimes you won't even know you have it. Even without symptoms, your doctor usually will be able to hear the abnormal sounds of the valve malfunctioning through his stethoscope. The murmurs are extra sounds in the heart, and they're due to the valve not opening or closing well, like a door that squeaks or sticks. The best way to diagnose valve disease is with an echocardiogram, which I'll discuss in Chapter 8.

The aortic valve is your biggest valve. It has three leaflets, and it's made of collagen, connective tissue, and elastic fibers. It is lined with endothelial cells, just like your arteries are. As we age, our aortic valves get stiffer. Sometimes this is due to high cholesterol or high blood pressure, so all the healthy lifestyle habits that protect your arteries also protect your aortic valve.

The most common valve problem is mitral valve prolapse. This is by far the cardiac problem I am most likely to see in my young women patients. The mitral valve is the valve between the left atrium and the left ventricle. It has two leaflets, so it looks like French doors. If you have mitral valve prolapse, it means the valve doesn't close correctly. There are different degrees of mitral valve prolapse, from mildly malfunctioning to severely malfunctioning. In mild cases, one of the "French door" flaps may swing slightly in the wrong direction, but you may never know you have it and it may not cause any problems. Sometimes the faulty valve can cause blood to leak abnormally into the left atrium from the left ventricle. The left ventricle then regurgitates the blood back into the left atrium.

In severe cases the little "French door" flaps can actually be broken. Severe mitral valve prolapse could lead to more severe problems, such as breaking off of the leaflets, leading to congestive heart failure or an infection of the valve, which can occur with any of the valves that are not functioning properly. Infection risk is the reason doctors often advise patients with mitral valve prolapse to take an antibiotic before dental work. The mouth has a lot of bacteria in it, and a mouth injury can send bacteria through the bloodstream. If the valves aren't working properly, this bacteria could get stuck on the valves, causing an infection. Recent guidelines suggest that antibiotics may not actually be necessary, but if you have mitral valve prolapse or any valve problem, talk to your doctor before you have dental work done.

Mitral valve prolapse is often associated with autonomic nervous system problems. We are not exactly sure why that is, but with mitral valve prolapse, autonomic nervous symptoms may develop, independent of the severity of the valve. Many times the autonomic problems manifest as electrical system issues like rapid heartbeats, palpitations, and difficulty exercising because of a rapid heart rate, as well as dizziness and passing out or the feeling of being lightheaded or fainting. An autonomic mismatch doesn't always have to be associated with mitral valve prolapse, although most of the time it is. Essentially what triggers an initially elevated heart rate leads to a blood pressure that plummets instead of increasing, and a heart rate that drops. Usually when the blood pressure drops, the heart rate speeds up in order to increase the volume of of blood delivered throughout the body and thereby maintain a normal blood pressure. When they drop in tandem, the result is often passing out or lightheadedness. This phenomenon will also happen in someone who has a primary autonomic dysfunction or POTS disease (postural orthostatic tachycardia syndrome). This mismatch, or autonomic imbalance, is what is seen when someone passes out from a pain response, is in an enclosed area that is hot, or is getting their blood drawn. It is called vasovagal syncope and it is the most common cause of passing out, especially in women.

Sometimes you can grow out of mitral valve prolapse. For some women, mitral valve prolapse actually improves after childbirth, during menopause, or as they age. This indicates a connection between mitral valve prolapse and hormones, although we aren't exactly sure what it is or how that might work. Mitral valve prolapse can also be inherited—I often see the problem in mothers and daughters.

Because of the link to the electrical system and the autonomic dysfunction leading to feeling faint, women with mitral valve prolapse often decide they have hypoglycemia (self-diagnosed). I see this a lot. They are actually experiencing mitral valve prolapse symptoms that they assume are blood sugar issues. However, the things that can help with blood sugar often do help mitral valve prolapse, like eating multiple times per day and staying well hydrated. This is because frequent snacks and plenty of fluids help keep the arteries filled, and this keeps the blood pressure up and the heart rate steady. This in turn can help with symptoms of lightheadedness or dizziness. I believe all women should keep themselves sustained, but if you have mitral valve prolapse, this is particularly important, and a possible treatment for the condition.

Now you know your heart a little bit better!

The purpose of this chapter is not to scare you or to get you obsessed, but only to help you get to know your heart as well as you know your other beloved parts. Clearly, there are more complexities to the story than I have explained to you; this is just an overview of what your heart does and how it works. If you are diagnosed with something heart-related, you can now understand what's actually going on in there.

Now you can also picture your heart in its perfectly healthy state, and that in itself is a heart-health strategy. Just like a coach will say to an Olympic athlete, "Picture what you need to do before you do it," visualizing your heart can help perfect its performance. Visualize your heart, with the doors opening and closing and the muscle squeezing. Picture the string of lights connecting the top and the bottom parts of the heart together through their electric pathways. See in your mind the miraculously efficient motor that keeps you vital, strong, healthy, young, vibrant, and alive. You are the operator, the maintenance person, the plumber, the mechanic. You make all the decisions about what your body will do to nurture your heart. You can be in charge of caring for your heart, because now you know how it works, and now you're motivated to care for it, pay attention to it, and live from it.

This Chapter, by Heart

♥ The heart is divided into four chambers, or "rooms," connected by valves, or "doors."

♥ Your heart contains four systems: the arteries, the muscle, the electrical system, and the valves.

♥ Heart problems may originate in any of the various systems or areas of the heart.

♥ Understanding what your heart looks like and how it works will help you appreciate the amazing machine inside your chest that keeps you alive. You want to do everything you can to keep it healthy and running strong!

CHAPTER FIVE

Why It's Up to You

Now that you are more intimately connected to the heart beating inside your own chest, I want to talk about something else you absolutely must know about your heart. I want to talk about why you might not get the kind of attention you really need.

I am sorry to be the one to explain this truth, but here it is. There is something going on behind the scenes in hospitals and doctors' offices that you need to know about because it affects you. It's this: Medicine is a business. Hospitals seek profits. They need profits to stay afloat, and they are expensive to run. They don't make money off of people who are well. They don't make money off of keeping people well. The dollars and cents come from people who are sick. That's the bottom line.

Sometimes, in order to be profitable, doctors may be encouraged to order unnecessary tests, and some doctors benefit directly from these tests. In some hospitals where doctors are salaried, their productivity measures are also based on how many patients they admit to the hospital and how many procedures are done.

This is why sometimes you hear those scary news reports about unnecessary procedures being done, or the closing of preventive pro-grams that lead to better health, such as cardiac rehabilitation. But even when there aren't news stories about these things, they happen. A hospital, and some doctors, may look for profits like a corporation. They look to the bottom line, and they evaluate what procedures and tests are most profitable, how long patients should be admitted based on a cost-benefit analysis, and whose care is getting reimbursed by insurance companies. Many if not most hospitals are driven to do business this way. It's just how businesses work. In these institutions, quantity is often the bottom line, and quality is the backup plan.

Of course, this isn't true of every hospital. Some centers receive grants and research dollars or are part of quality control or massive health-care initiatives to provide the best care for their patients, with discharge planning to prevent readmission and promote the optimum health for their patients. Some institutions are paving the way to help patients better take care of themselves. But here is the real bottom line: Prevention isn't profitable.

Preventive programs in hospitals, like cardiac rehabilitation or wellness programs, don't get nearly as much funding as programs for treating diseases, because they don't bring in as much money for the hospital, so patients who are seeking out prevention might have a hard time actually getting it. There are such things as annual well-ness checkups covered by insurance, but comprehensive wellness pro-grams in hospitals are simply hard to find. Putting in stents and performing open-heart surgeries generate revenue. Any revenue gen-erated by providing a place for people to work out or learn about healthy eating or stress management can't compare.

It makes perfect sense from a business standpoint. How can a business support the programs that don't bring in any money? But in the business of medicine, sometimes the patients get forgotten. That's why it is so important for you to empower yourself. You need to take control of your self-care. It's the only real way, and it's good business for *you* because when you get sick, you have to pay the bills.

It's not that the health-care system doesn't *want* you to be well, but they are in the business of treating those who are sick. This is just one major reason why you must know that your health, your heart, and your vitality are *up to you.* Nobody else is looking out for it. A hospital is immersed in paying its own bills, negotiating with the insurance companies, and haggling over reimbursement rates. Fortunately, things are changing, with issues like "pay per performance" and with doctors and hospitals being held accountable for health outcomes, and with initiatives to prevent hospital readmissions. But change is slow, and if you are a business, of course profit is the bottom line.

Prevention has traditionally not been the focus in medical school, so when your doctor doesn't know the best fats for you to eat or which vitamins are recommended, try not to get too upset. It just hasn't been part of the curriculum. We have been a culture of reactive, not preventive, medicine. Doctors know more about doing expensive medical procedures than how to prescribe a heart-healthy diet.

Wellness is *your* business. The only person who can be truly interested in your wellness—who has a *vested interest* in your wellness—is you.

Now, I do have to say that plenty of expensive medical tests and procedures *are often justified,* and as a patient, you aren't usually in a position to judge whether you really need an angiogram or not. If your doctor tells you to get one, you probably should do it, but seek out a second opinion if you feel uncomfortable. None of this will be an issue, though, if you avoid getting sick in the first place. Take care of your own bottom line, not the hospital's or the doctor's. To do this, you need to stay well.

You won't be alone in your efforts at prevention. The American Heart Association's Go Red For Women campaign is a true preventive effort, educating and empowering women to take care of their health. The Go Red "Know Your Numbers" initiative reminds women that prevention is in their hands. I'm a spokesperson for this campaign, with a great passion for their mission, as Going Red is all about prevention and self-empowerment. Women are drawn to Go Red events because many have been let down by the medical community in terms of getting diagnosed, getting proper treatment, or receiving preventative advice.

If your hospital has a center for women's health, a diabetes prevention program, or a women and heart disease program, then by all means take advantage of it, and make it known to the hospital that you support these types of programs.

Recently, another doctor pulled me aside and said, "Okay, tell me the truth. This whole 'women and heart disease thing,' it's just a marketing ploy, right?" I was stunned into silence. And then I let him have it. When I'm angry, I become like a walking encyclopedia. Every study I'd ever read, every female victim of heart disease I'd ever known, it all came pouring out of me. Finally, all I could say was, "Do you have any more questions?"

Perhaps I overreacted (I suspect as much from the startled look on his face!). But perhaps I didn't, because this doctor genuinely did not believe that heart disease is a legitimate problem that is distinct and separate in women, even though we know for a fact it is the number-one killer of women, appears differently in women, and is harder to diagnose in women. He didn't know it or believe it, nor did he see why it was really important. And he was a doctor. He could be your doctor.

Just the other day as I was walking through the hospital, I passed a room and I heard a doctor say, "If you can't trust your doctor, who can you trust?" Even as a doctor myself, I had to laugh out loud at this. I wanted to step into the room and look right at that patient and say, "Yourself! That's who you can trust if you can't trust your doctor!"

I wish doctors knew everything and had crystal balls that could show them exactly what is wrong with you. I wish they had a pill to solve every problem. I'm sorry to say they do not. We do not.

So in this chapter, I want to look into what I will charitably call this "situation," because I want to show you exactly why doctors may not take your heart symptoms seriously, why they may misdiagnose you, and why it isn't really in their best interests to change. When you understand the reasons, you'll understand the urgency. And then maybe we can make some progress.

You Don't Look Sick

When you walk in the door and you are a young and vibrant-looking woman, the initial response from your doctor is going to be that your heart is fine. You don't look sick, so chances are you aren't sick. That's a common misconception.

Doctors are taught to evaluate a patient's vitality in a certain way, and a person with serious heart disease usually looks sick. In my office, however, I look for a little bit more than the obvious. I assess vitality, and it's obvious to me when a patient doesn't have it.

One of the ways I do this is to assess vanity. If a patient is well-groomed and paying attention to her appearance, I suspect she isn't feeling too bad. When she is obviously letting things slip, that's a red flag to me. Of course, this isn't always true—I've had very well-groomed women come into my office who were very ill—but it can be a clue. In fact, whenever I would be doing rounds in the hospital, checking up on patients in recovery, I would employ what I called the Lipstick Test. When a patient had actually put on lipstick, I knew she was almost ready to go home.

But the signs of lost vitality can be even more subtle. (And maybe you never wear lipstick!) Just because you look fabulous doesn't mean heart disease isn't gaining a foothold. You may not be sick *right now*, but that doesn't mean you aren't headed down that road. Your doctor can't see it, even though you might be feeling it manifesting in vague aches and pains, heart flutters and occasional dizziness or nausea, or that general frustrating feeling that something is wrong, even though you can't quite put a well-manicured finger on it.

But your doctor just sees what's in front of him. He reads the lab reports. He listens to your heart. And if everything looks fine, or mostly fine, he is likely to tell you that you are fine and send you on your merry way.

Your doctor won't begin to suspect you are having a health problem until he gets to know you. He has to be aware of who he is talking to. Otherwise he won't have a clear understanding of your risk. He won't see that you need information *now*, that you need a treatment plan *now*, before you look sick, before you come in with your vitality sapped, before you've painstakingly made it through menopause and have high cholesterol, high blood pressure, and diabetes. Then it will be obvious, but do you want to wait until then to try to figure out how you got there? Of course not, if you can avoid ever going there in the first place.

You're a Woman

It's not that doctors don't understand you. It's just that they don't . . . well, they don't understand *you*.

Not only are you completely individual and not necessarily like anybody in any study on which they base their treatment, but you are a woman, and when it comes to heart disease, not to mention your position in society, doctors (including female doctors) don't always know what to make of you. Because heart studies often don't include women and heart symptoms aren't always obvious in women, your symptoms might seem mysterious. You require more guesswork, more extrapolation. You are *confusing*.

You might also be more likely than a man to attribute your symptoms to stress, thereby dismissing them. This is a mistake! You are also much more likely to tell your doctor that it might be "all in my head." Please don't utter those words in a doctor's office, I beg of you! When you say that to a doctor, he may just assume you are correct, and that it really *is* all in your head. He may not look as carefully. He may not take you as seriously. So please, watch what you say. Stick to a clear explanation of your symptoms and avoid making judgments about what you think is or is not wrong with you. Don't let the fear of inconveniencing the doctor or fear of sounding like a hypochondriac keep you from explaining how you really feel. (I'll talk a lot more about how to talk to your doctor in Chapter 6.)

On top of all that, at least culturally speaking, you're actually acting more like a man these last few decades. Sort of. You live a more active and stressful life in the world, you have more power, but you still have those unmanly heart symptoms. Doctors do the best they can to assess your symptoms, but they aren't always going to get it right.

I want to talk a little more about this "acting like a man" business, because I think it is very important for women to understand where this has put us in terms of not only the medical profession but how it affects our hearts. In 2009, journalist Maria Shriver and the Center for American Progress published a document called *The Shriver Report: A Woman's Nation Changes Everything*. This report took a close look at the role of working women in the United States and what being a working mother means today. The report reveals that women now hold half of all jobs but are still primarily responsible for taking care of the home and children, even though most jobs do not make allowances for this need. The new workforce is made up of breadwinning moms who are trying to do it all: financially support the family, emotionally support the family, take care of the kids, and try to stay healthy (that's typically last on the list).

A 2009 poll, reported on in *The Shriver Report*, asked households in which both partners work whether the woman takes on more responsibilities for the home and family than her male partner. The results: 85 percent of the women said yes, they do take on more of the responsibilities, and 67 percent of the men agreed that this was true. All this extra responsibility is stressful. Men and women don't parcel out our home-vs.-work duties like we used to. Women are trying to do it all. But this isn't always possible.

Unfortunately, much of the world isn't set up to foster the working mother, and yet most of us are doing it anyway, struggling along, making up the rules as we go. Sometimes we feel powerful and strong, but sometimes we feel like we're falling apart. There is no playbook, or set of rules, for this new generation of women. We are learning as we go. We're still working out how to do it all, let alone how to do it well.

When I started out in medicine, I was young, and I looked even younger than my actual age. I was chipper, enthusiastic, and willing to do my best. I was an extremely hard worker, but I definitely wasn't trying to be a man. I was always a girly-girl. I'm all about collecting cute bras, not burning them.

On the first day of my internship, I went to work. I'd laid out my work clothes the night before so that I wouldn't be too stressed in the morning deciding what to wear. I put out a skirt and a sweater, and the next morning I put them on and I went to work. Normal, right?

When I got to the hospital and we started rounds, I had my list of things to do, and as I was leaning over a chart reading my list, I noticed a nurse staring at me.

"Hi?"

She just looked at me. Then she said, in a dry and cynical voice, if I recall correctly, "If you ever want to be taken seriously, never wear a skirt to work."

That was the last day that I wore a skirt to work for many years.

The skirt became a symbol in my mind. I had assumed I could be myself, and also be a doctor, but day in and day out, in the trenches of my job, it often felt like that was going to be an impossible combination. Being a woman isn't necessarily part of the equation in the man's world of conventional medicine. Throughout my career, I've had to struggle every step of the way to do what I thought was right, to exercise my female point of view, to champion prevention, to do only the tests I thought were legitimately necessary, and to be who I really am in the workplace. In the world of professional medicine, I've always received the subtle, or not-so-subtle, message that these beliefs of mine were not as relevant, or as critical, as the mainstream views of patching up what has already gone wrong.

This isn't only about medicine. I know many women in many professions who are trying to change the world and often meet with resistance. It's not just me. But I've finally reached the point in my career when I can smile as I put a dress on to go to work, because I made the decision to be myself rather than the person I felt pressured to be. I don't feel like I have to prove myself anymore, at least not through my clothing choices. Yes, now that I am more senior in my field than I used to be, on that day, I decided it was time to wear a dress to work. I had already earned respect for the work I was doing, so it shouldn't matter what I was wearing. We've all made some progress, and women are more accepted in every profession than they ever have been before, but the struggle is not over.

Some of that struggle is internal. I fight myself much less now than when I was a "baby" doctor, new to the field, but I still struggle with juggling career and family and being a woman in a world that's largely still male-dominated and -oriented. We all do.

I believe this is part of what hurts women's hearts. If you can't be you, stay you, maintain yourself, and always, first and foremost, take care of your heart and put yourself first, then your heart will suffer.

There might not be a study that proves this very specific thing, but I know from decades of experience that it's true. When I say, "Live from the heart," I'm saying, "Live from that place of who you are." It's not about wearing pants or a skirt and it's not about conforming to what others think. It's about really understanding your best qualities and letting them shine. Know who you are and the rest will follow.

Still, the fact remains that the world is still largely constructed around the needs, temperaments, and professional lives of men, and yet women are working in it, participating in it, side by side with men. Sometimes that works for us, and sometimes it doesn't. Another quote from *The Shriver Report*: "Even if our parents didn't call themselves feminists, we, the daughters of the 1980s and 1990s, were raised with a new and improved edict of equality. You can do anything you want to do, just like your brothers." What they didn't tell us was that for us it would be harder than it was for our brothers.

This reality has two results: It stresses our hearts, so we are having more heart problems than we used to have. Doctors don't expect that, so they don't always see it in time. And research hasn't caught up to the heart problems that have grown out of this new paradigm. Public health statistics are there, but they don't necessarily apply to *you*.

You Are Not the Focus of the Primary Research Studies

Over the past few decades, there have been several comprehensive and crucial studies and initiatives that have helped cardiologists define the most common risk factors for heart disease in the general population. This is a good thing. It has saved many lives. (For the rest of this chapter, I talk about "risk factors" in terms of public health, but remember, when a so-called risk factor applies to you personally, that is what I call a Heart Throb.)

When I look back over the evolution of heart disease treatment, there are four studies, scores, or initiatives that have been landmarks along the way that I want you to understand: the Framingham Heart Study, the Reynolds Risk Score, the Interheart Study, and an action plan developed by the American Heart Association called the Simple Seven. These studies, scores, and initiatives represent how the medical profession has evolved to determine your risk factors for heart disease. For many years, the first study I'm going to tell you about, the Framingham Heart Study, has been used to determine whether someone is at risk for heart disease and to decide on diagnostic procedures and treatment plans. In fact, this is what the insurance companies use to determine if they will approve a test that your doctor might have ordered.

I use the information we've learned from these studies and initiatives in my practice every day, and any one or more of them are likely to influence how doctors will evaluate *your* risk of heart disease and how they will diagnose *your* symptoms. But the problem with these studies is that they aren't comprehensive enough. Let's consider why.

THE FRAMINGHAM HEART STUDY

It all started in a small town called Framingham, Massachusetts, in 1948. When I imagine Framingham, I see one of those little Christmas villages with white picket fences and little snow-capped roofs. It's where men went to work in the morning after their wives made them a hearty breakfast of eggs, bacon, pancakes, and freshly squeezed orange juice. The wives mostly stayed home, took care of the house, then met their husbands at the door with slippers, a cigar, and a shot of Scotch. At least that's how I picture it. I think of those old black-and-white television shows, like *Father Knows Best* or *Leave It to Beaver*. I think of a life completely unlike the one most of us live today.

I don't know about you, but I don't have a white picket fence, I don't cook breakfast, and hell, I don't even have the husband anymore. I'm the one who goes off to work in the morning. The reality that the Framingham study is based on is completely foreign to me, and probably to you too.

Still, this was the scene for a massive study on heart health and risk factors that extended from 1948 to 1961. The residents of this town were analyzed, and then their offspring were analyzed, and we found out a lot of information. To summarize, we found out that your age, gender, total cholesterol, HDL (the so-called good) cholesterol, smoking status, and systolic blood pressure are the primary factors that put people at risk for heart disease.

Researchers used this information to develop the Framingham Risk Analysis, a simple tool that can evaluate someone's heart disease risk based on the factors that are most likely to lead to heart disease in the general population. By looking at these factors alone, we can predict, with pretty great accuracy, who will and who will not have a heart attack in the next ten years. This has helped a lot of people. It has saved lives.

The problem is with heart patients who have heart attacks *despite* the odds as calculated by the Framingham Risk Analysis. For example, young women who have high levels of naturally occurring estrogen tend to have very high levels of HDL cholesterol. That's the good cholesterol that tends to be protective. So for those young women, according to the Framingham Risk Analysis, their heart disease risk is automatically low, due to their gender, age, and HDL level. Yet this is the very population in which we are seeing an increased incidence of heart disease. Framingham doesn't explain this.

THE REYNOLDS HEART STUDY

The Reynolds Heart Study is another significant landmark in the history of cardiology. The Reynolds Heart Study was a ten-year study that started in September 1992. Although it included both men and women, the number of women in the study was significantly higher than in other studies up to that point. The Reynolds Heart Study included 24,000 women 45 years and older, and it found that up to 20 percent of all coronary events were missed by doctors who used the Framingham Risk Analysis to evaluate risk. Why were these women having heart attacks? The researchers wanted to find the missing elements, the disconnect between Framingham and their results.

This became the Reynolds Heart Study, and it looked at a number of additional risk factors to see if these women had any signs of an impending coronary event. Indeed, they did have some other risk factors the Framingham Risk Analysis doesn't consider, like a family history of heart disease, inflammation, an elevated hemoglobin A1C (a test for diabetes), and more specific cholesterol measurements, like apolipoprotein B. The Reynolds Heart Study categorized these additional risks and found that when applied to a large group of women, this new risk assessment model was able to catch more at-risk women than the Framingham Risk Analysis. So that was progress!

THE INTERHEART STUDY

Another significant model for risk assessment is based on a major study conducted in 2004 called the Interheart Study, which gave us even more information. This study identified nine risk factors that account for a full 90 percent of heart attacks:

- An abnormal apolipoprotein B/apolipoprotein A-1 ratio (this involves the apolipoprotein B we talked about in the Heart Throbs chapter—it is the protein carrier for the worst kind of cholesterol)
- Smoking
- Diabetes

- Hypertension (high blood pressure)

- Abdominal obesity

- Psychosocial risk factors (things like depression, anxiety, hostility, and stress)

- Lack of daily fruit and vegetable consumption

- Lack of exercise

- Excessive alcohol consumption

This study was particularly useful for assessing general risk because the risk factors it included were the same in almost every geographic region and racial or ethnic group worldwide, and also the same in men and women. It was the first one to analyze behaviors like diet and exercise, alcohol intake, and psychosocial issues. *Aha . . .* instead of just numbers, these studies were starting to look like they described actual people!

THE SIMPLE SEVEN

Finally, the American Heart Association recently set a very important goal. By the year 2020, they want to improve the cardiovascular health of all Americans by 20 percent and reduce deaths from cardiovascular disease and stroke by 20 percent. In order to help make this happen, they developed a set of Impact Goals for the year 2020. This wasn't simply a study but an action plan to jump in and try to fix the problem of heart disease. They targeted four health behaviors and three health factors that we can all put into action to stop the disease process before it starts or arrest it at an early stage. These behaviors and factors are controllable, and they will, *in almost all cases,* keep the heart healthy well into old age. According to the research behind these goals, if you incorporate just five of them, you'll have a 78 percent lower risk of death from any cause and an 88 percent lower risk of death from cardiovascular disease. Here we had an action plan, a true evolution.

AHA Life's Simple Seven

1. Don't smoke.
2. Maintain a healthy weight.
3. Exercise regularly.
4. Eat a healthy diet.
5. Maintain a total cholesterol level of less than 200.
6. Maintain blood pressure of less than 120/80.
7. Maintain a fasting blood sugar level of 100 mg/dL or less.

So all of this is fantastic and fabulous and lifesaving, but what does it all mean for you? Remember, we're talking about *you*, not statistics, not public health, not generalized risk.

When your doctor takes your history or examines you to determine whether or not you might be at risk for the number-one cause of death in the United States, he is most likely going to be thinking about the Framingham Risk Analysis, even though it's the oldest and least comprehensive, and caters least to women's risk. It's still the one many doctors and insurance companies default to when analyzing risk.

But if you don't fit the profile, as you sit there in a cold, bright office in a flimsy gown wondering what the verdict is, or why you're having chest pains or palpitations or dizziness or fatigue or anxiety or nausea or just a feeling that something is wrong, then your doctor might not catch what's going on. You have the right to say, "What if it's heart disease?" But you might not think to say it if you yourself don't understand that you are at risk, and exactly *how* you are at risk.

You Are Not a Number

It all comes down to this simple fact: You are not a risk-benefit analysis. You are a person, with a risk profile as individual as you are, and nobody can possibly know you better than you know yourself.

You have a family history. You have lifestyle habits. Some that you don't check off on the health assessment form. Some that you keep secret.

You also have a heart unlike anyone else's. I really don't know anyone or have any patients that fit into the *Father Knows Best* paradigm that I associate with the Framingham Heart Study, so how could I possibly simply rely on that to help me figure out the risk in my women patients as they live today? I can't, because every one of my patients is unique. But that is what doctors have been trained to do. That's why you have to know yourself. That is why I wanted you to think about the Heart Throbs in such a personal way.

Knowing your tendencies, your strengths, and your weaknesses, and how the medical profession is likely to respond to you and your apparent risk profile, is entirely up to you. Who you are determines where you go next, what you do for yourself, and what kind of care you demand. In my mind, it's simple. Know who you are and empower yourself to change your life now, before it's too late. Only you can take the first step. Only you can seek out the care and support you need. This is doable. I've seen it happen over and over again. You can change your path, and you must, or those statistics about increasing heart disease in women are only going to get worse. You could become a statistic. Or you could help to forge a path toward a new statistic, where heart disease is *no longer* the number-one killer of women.

Let's make a change, one heart at a time. Let's start with yours.

This Chapter, by Heart

♥ Prevention isn't taught and isn't profitable, so your doctor may not know much about it and hospitals don't prioritize funding for programs that promote it.

♥ In many ways, the world is still organized around the needs of men. As women try to fit in and excel in that world, they are still trying to figure out how to make that work. This is stressful and could be one cause for the increase in heart disease in younger women.

♥ Doctors tend to misdiagnose or underdiagnose heart disease in women because the symptoms tend to be more vague and unclear than they are in men, and the diagnostic tests may not always be accurate.

♥ If you want to avoid ever having heart symptoms that require diagnosis and treatment in a hospital, you have to take responsibility for your own health and implement preventive practices.

CHAPTER SIX

Inside the Office:
The Art and Challenge of
Communicating with Doctors

Doctors aren't all alike. Some are particularly good at communicating, and others most definitely are not. Communication skills, or lack thereof, are probably the number-one reason people say "I love my doctor" or "I can't stand my doctor." Sometimes we call this "bedside manner," but you don't have to be in a bed to experience a doctor's skill with it, or lack of it.

When doctors don't communicate well, this can cause a lot of problems for patients—not just in feeling discarded or not listened to, but even in their ultimate diagnosis and in how they comprehend how to manage their medical problems.

But here's the thing—as much as doctors need to work on their communication skills (and they do!), you can do a lot to improve the situation. I'm not saying it's all up to you—communication is a two-way street—but in this chapter, I'm going to talk about how you can communicate better with your doctor, and possibly even break down some of the barriers that have existed between you.

Time Issues

The first thing you should know is that most doctors allot fifteen minutes per patient. The goal is to get down to the problem as quickly as possible so it can be fixed as quickly as possible. It's not the doctor's fault. Today doctors have huge demands on their time, dealing with health insurance companies and fitting in all the patients they are required to see. That means you don't have long to state your case, and your doctor doesn't have long to review it.

The first time I met my patient Maddy, she came into my office carrying a huge white three-ring binder. It was filled with hundreds of pages: lab reports, patient records, Internet pages printed out, and e-mails from doctors and people who weren't doctors but thought they knew what was wrong with her. The pages were covered with sticky notes and tags, and many of the pages had passages highlighted or circled in red, with arrows and exclamation points. It was all organized with dividers and tags according to what problems she thought she probably had.

"Please tell me you haven't been pushing that binder on every doctor you see," I said.

Her eyes widened. "I've shown it to everyone," she said.

Maddy had been through a lot. She was 36 years old, married with no children, and she was a teacher. The reason she'd been to so many doctors was that she kept fainting—in Bloomingdale's, on the subway a couple of times, in school. She came to see me for a second opinion because somewhere along the way, during a succession of visits to multiple different specialists, someone had recommended she get a pacemaker. Sometimes a pacemaker is the best treatment for fainting, but I wasn't sure that a pacemaker would ultimately be the right solution for her. When I examined her, I kept asking her questions, and she kept wanting to show me her binder. There was no way I had time to go through that binder, and I was more interested in her story—what she had to tell me right then and there. She wanted to talk about her theories and what every doctor had said before, and what every magazine, website, and article she found also said. That binder was beyond a collection of medical records. It was an encyclopedia of medical frustration.

"Put away the binder," I said. "Just tell me your story."

Maddy had a difficult problem that wasn't easily diagnosed. When doctors failed to help her, she began to compile information. She got opinions from everyone. She researched her symptoms on the Internet and formed theories about what might be wrong with her. After all, the doctors weren't figuring it out, right? Somebody had to do it, and Maddy wanted to take her health care into her own hands, just as I tell my patients to do.

I understood the binder. Maddy was trying to piece together her own story to help the doctors figure it out. *She was trying to help them help her.* But it wasn't working because the important stuff—the medical records and the test results—were buried under pages and pages of information that wasn't helping anyone.

Maddy's approach was hindering communication. I understood her frustration, but her particular efforts to help herself weren't helping, and her research efforts were only pushing doctors away. So I went back to her story, and I asked her again: What happens before and after you pass out?

It turned out that right before she passed out, every single time, she had severe stomach cramps and diarrhea. She'd already seen a gastroenterologist for the stomach issues, a neurologist for headaches, and a cardiologist for palpitations, but nobody had put all the pieces together. After tracking her particular symptoms, she tried a gluten-free diet and her fainting reduced significantly. Her underlying anxiety and fear over her illness was managed, and she started becoming healthier and stronger. Maddy never actually got a firm diagnosis, but the fainting was obviously related to her gastrointestinal issues, not to her heart, and what I believe was an autonomic nervous system dysfunction that was triggered by her GI issues. When she healed her gut, her problem resolved.

Doctors do need to see your tests and your previous diagnoses, but in Maddy's case, I didn't need to see the binder. I just needed to hear her story, and that's what your doctor needs too. Give him the bottom line, tell him where you are *now*, and go from there.

Your Heart

One of the barriers to doctor-patient communication is actually poor doctor-to-doctor communication. Unless there is a shared electronic medical record, the doctor you see has no way to know about your previous diagnoses and test results *unless you provide them.* Even if you tell Doctor X that you already saw Doctor Y, do you think they are going to meet over cocktails to discuss your case? I can assure you they are not. They don't have time, and doctors are horrendously bad about conferring anyway. Take this common communication glitch into your own hands and keep copies of your records. When you get referred to a specialist or seek a second opinion, your doctor won't have to duplicate tests or start at square one when another doctor has already gotten you to square six.

What Your Doctor Needs to Know

Your doctor speaks a special language, and he spent a lot of time learning how to speak it. The language of medicine took that doctor four years of medical school, four years of residency, and maybe four more years of fellowship to master.

Patients, on the other hand, speak in laymen's terms. They can be incredibly articulate, but they cannot speak the language of medicine as fluently as a doctor. This is one of the main reasons doctors and patients often fail to communicate well. When patients try to speak the language of medicine (by, for example, diagnosing themselves or using medical terms to describe their symptoms), the message may get lost. The doctor may not understand, because the patient doesn't really know how to use the language correctly, or the doctor may even be offended because the patient is treading on his toes. Wrong or right, this can happen.

You should not be expected to speak the language of medicine. In fact, somewhat like a Parisian waiter, the doctor may not want you to even try to speak his language. However, that Parisian waiter had better speak English if he's going to pooh-pooh your French, and your doctor needs to be able to hear you if he wants to translate what you say into the language of medicine. You can make this easier on your doctor by communicating in a very particular way.

Don't worry, I'll get to doctors and their issues soon enough, but you can do more about your own communication than you can about theirs, so let's start with you. By no means am I pointing a finger at you. I just want to give you things to do. You're reading this book and the doctors aren't. Believe me, I know how difficult doctors can be! But this is your book, and it's meant to give you action steps.

Doctors want to know if you have a diagnosis, and they do want to see your medical records. Your medical records are important, that giant binder notwithstanding. Doctors need to see them. They don't want to start from scratch if another doctor has already run tests or even diagnosed you, and they should know if you are seeking out a first opinion from them or a second. (Or a third.) What doctors do not want is for you to interpret the tests for them or offer your own diagnosis in the absence of a diagnosis from a doctor. The fact is that you are (probably) not a doctor, and even if you are, you need someone objective when the patient is you. Yes, you know more than a doctor about how you feel, but your doctor's specialty is diagnosing and treating disease. This is an important distinction. Your doctor shouldn't tell you how to feel, and you shouldn't tell your doctor what you think your diagnosis is.

Doctors want to hear your symptoms. Better yet, they want a timeline of your symptoms. In other words, they want the story. Don't be afraid to tell your doctor what is bothering you. I needed to hear from Maddy, "I pass out." I needed to know that of all the symptoms she was having, this one was disrupting her life the most. And I needed her to answer my questions about that symptom so I could form my own theory. That's why she came to me.

The reason doctors need a clear explanation of your symptoms is that they have been trained to diagnose you in a very particular way. It's a method that allows us to put together a *differential diagnosis*, or a list of possible diagnoses. Understanding how this works can help you to understand what information your doctor needs from you and what information will just confuse the issue.

To help you understand how this works, I'll explain the art of taking a good medical history. This is a crucial class in medical school and my explanation of it here is extrapolated from a textbook I have from when I was a first-year medical student. It explains the physical exam and the art of diagnosis via taking a patient's history. This is how it works:

- First, you ask for a chief complaint.

- Then you ask for the onset, frequency, and duration of the complaint.

- Then you ask for the progression.

- Then you ask if there is anything that makes it better or worse.

- What seems to be associated with the symptom?

- What time of day does it happen?

If the symptom is pain-related, then the next series of questions is about the location and quality of the pain:

- Does it radiate?

- How severe is it on a scale of 1 to 10?

- When does it start?

- How long does it last?

- What setting are you in when it happens?

This is how doctors have learned how to listen, so when you start naming diseases instead of symptoms, your doctor can't explore the possibilities the way they've been trained to do. Because a doctor is focused on making a differential diagnosis, your own personal theories on your diagnosis are not helpful. When you understand this, you will see why it's not a good idea to add extra, unnecessary information. "I have chest pain" is helpful. "I think I have angina" is not helpful. I understand why so many patients do this: With the popularization of online health websites and all those morning shows and "medical mystery" shows that "help" you figure out exactly what you think you've got, the doctor-patient relationship has changed. Patients not only know more than they used to about their own health, they sometimes think they know more than they really know. Again, *you know your body*. You know your symptoms. You might have theories about what's wrong with you, *and they might be right*. But diagnosis is your doctor's job, and your doctor has access to more information about what your symptoms might mean than you do. More information than that morning show. More information than the Internet. And more experience too. So if you go to a doctor, it only makes sense to step back a bit and let him do his job. Believe it or not, most of them like their jobs, and part of the fun of it is figuring out what is wrong and then doing something to help!

A doctor can only do what he knows best, so let's all open the lines of communication and stick to the facts, and then we'll all be working from the same rulebook and we can get you the best medical care and attention you need. Tell your story right away, so you can be heard. I think if that happened more often, I wouldn't hear from so many of my patients, "Why didn't I know that?" or "Why didn't anyone tell me that?"

Listen, I know that it's scary when you think you might have something wrong with you and you feel like nobody can figure out what it is. That's how Maddy felt. We're constantly exposed to stories that tell us the most horrible things about health. We get scared that such a thing will happen to us. I understand that. I know that when you go to the doctor, you might already be in an emotionally charged place, and that can make it difficult to stick to the facts and be calm and clear. You can even reveal your anxiety—tell your doctor that your best friend dropped dead of a heart attack at 50 years old and you want to make sure that doesn't happen to you. That's helpful information because it tells the doctor what you are looking for from him.

Heart Sense

When it comes to researching your health on the Internet, stick to the sites of well-established organizations, particularly nonprofit foundations that represent the disease state that is relevant to you. These organizations aren't making any money, so they don't have an agenda. They are the most likely to give you unbiased but reliable information and to foster groups of people in a similar situation. Find websites that aren't selling you products. Look for those that are providing you credible information. Avoid profit-driven organizations, and also avoid putting too much stock in sites designed by nonmedical professionals, even those that don't have something to sell. There is a lot of bad information on the Internet.

Also remember that even the best website cannot provide you with a diagnosis. I've seen people confidently telling other people their diagnoses, which they've decided are accurate based on online research, even though there are no such diagnoses in their medical records. Maybe they are right, but what are the consequences of being wrong? Diagnosing yourself can result in misrepresenting symptoms to your doctor, and then you might not get an accurate diagnosis after all, so be careful. Learn, but don't assume.

Doctors only want to hear your most important symptoms. One of the things I can personally attest to that makes a relationship with a patient difficult is when that person comes in with nine million symptoms, along with a reason they've already decided is the cause of each symptom. Like, "I have a twinging in my arm, and I think it's because my calcium's low because I read that on the Internet. And I also have headaches and fatigue, so I think I have fibromyalgia. And my stomach is upset a lot, which is probably IBS. But I wonder if I might have celiac disease because sometimes I'm nauseated after I eat bread. That might also be why I'm gaining too much weight, because although the Internet says that it's more common to lose weight with celiac disease, I've talked to a lot of people on this autoimmune forum who said they are overweight. Do you think I could have lupus?"

My first thought when I hear this is, "Breathe. Just breathe."

This is why it benefits you to get your symptom priorities in order. Pick your most bothersome symptoms—the ones that seem the most severe to you or that impact your quality of life the most. Stick to three or four, possibly five. No more. In most cases, all your other symptoms are caused by whatever is causing the main symptoms anyway. Then, if your doctor asks you, through the process of forming the differential diagnosis, "Do you also have this, or this, or that?" you can confidently answer "Yes" or "No."

Another thing that can happen is that I'll be with a patient talking through everything, and when we are done, I'll turn the doorknob to leave the office and they'll say, "Oh, by the way, did I tell you that I have chest pain when I walk?" Now, this is a serious concern and justifies testing, and I think, "Whoa, you're just telling me this now? You are mentioning your chest pain to the cardiologist as an afterthought?"

In journalism they would call this "burying the lede." Give your doctor the front-page headlines. "I have chest pain and nausea." "I keep fainting." "I'm short of breath." "I have jaw pain and back pain when I walk, but it stops when I rest."

Doctors don't want or need to hear a thousand symptoms, but we do need to know all the relevant background. Not what you *think* is wrong, but what has already actually happened to you. That includes diseases or surgeries or accidents you had, even as a child. I had a young patient who had pulmonary stenosis—a too-tight heart valve—as a baby, which was surgically repaired. When she started to experience shortness of breath, extreme fatigue, and a feeling of unwellness at 26 years old, some doctors told her it wasn't related to her heart, but they didn't know her pediatric history. It turned out that she needed a valve replacement, but without the surgical information about her valve repair, her doctors didn't have a chance of getting it right. So give us the facts!

Also be sure to mention the relevant symptoms according to what specialist you are seeing. If you are seeing a cardiologist, talk about your heart symptoms. Don't mention how you twisted your ankle or how you are having chronic diarrhea or headaches. If your doctor then asks, through the process of trying to put together a differential diagnosis, if you are having any gastrointestinal problems or headaches, then certainly provide that information, but don't lead with it.

I do understand that sometimes you just don't have the words. You don't completely know how you feel, or you don't know how to verbalize it. You might forget things that happened to you as a child. You might leave out something important. You might want to tell your story in a way that isn't as helpful for your doctor. It happens, and nobody expects you to be perfect. Just try your best, knowing what you now know.

Doctors need to know the truth. The whole truth. About seven years ago, I had a patient who was 34 years old. She was thin, ate well, and had extremely high blood pressure. She had no family history of heart disease and her high blood pressure was a complete mystery. I took care of her for three years, and I just couldn't figure out what could be causing her strange condition. I kept saying to her, "This isn't normal. I don't know what's happening. What are you doing?"

"Nothing, nothing, I swear!" she said to me, again and again.

Then one Monday morning she came in to my office and she said, "I need to tell you something. I'm really sorry. I'm an alcoholic, and I'm going into rehab."

Excuse me? *Excuse me?* I couldn't believe what I was hearing. All along she had known exactly why her blood pressure was so high. But she wasn't about to tell me.

I understand why, of course. She didn't want to admit to her problem. She didn't want to think that was the reason. But it was. Excessive alcohol consumption raises your blood pressure, sometimes dangerously. Four years later, she's sober and we laugh about it. She's a new person and her life is much better. But my point, of course, is that if you want your doctor to do the best possible job he can to help you, *you have to give him all the information.*

We aren't mind readers. We can't conjure up miracle diagnoses with major pieces of the puzzle missing. So please, please, give us the information. When it says on that form you fill out, "How many drinks per week," don't put "three" when the truth is "thirty."

Yes, we might tell you to stop doing what you are doing, but we are only doing this because we know it will help you, and you came to us to help you. Right? And no, we won't tell your mother.

Doctors want to answer your questions. What they don't want is to be lectured or tested or challenged or directed or told what to do. Maybe this isn't the best of a doctor's qualities, but nobody really likes these things, so why should doctors?

I had a patient with a very difficult autoimmune disease, and she was having a lot of communication issues with her rheumatologist. I could tell by the way she described their conversations to me that he felt very challenged by her mode of communication.

This wasn't her fault. She was frustrated because nobody could diagnose her, and she kept pushing him for a diagnosis he couldn't give. She was also doing it in a particular way that was setting him off. I know this doctor, and I know how he thinks, and he might not be the easiest guy to get along with, but he's also brilliant, and I wouldn't want her seeing anyone else. She just didn't know that she was pushing his buttons.

This is what I said to her: *Try this experiment: When you speak to him, only ask him questions. Don't tell him anything.*

Several months later, she called me in my office and she told me she couldn't believe the difference. "He's helping me! We're talking!" she said.

Your doctor studied hard for a long time to get good at what he does, and if you come in and challenge him or try to get him to just tell you what you want to hear, or worse yet, say something like "There's a doctor at Columbia who said I have X, so you must be wrong," then of course he's going to get annoyed with you. He might be tempted to say, "Dude, then go to Columbia! There's the door!" I've had patients who were clearly testing me or challenging me or implying that I didn't know what they knew or what other doctors knew or as much as I should know. Nobody likes that. It's no way to get the best from a doctor.

But when a patient asks me questions? Wants my help? I will give her everything I've got.

When you get confused or upset about communication, it's important to remember what you really want out of the interaction with your doctor. You want to know what's going to happen to you, plain and simple, right? So ask *that*. If you are pushing for a diagnosis and you aren't getting it, push for the thing you *really* want. Ask your doctor: What happens to people like me who are experiencing these symptoms?

There are doctors, and many other people, who are, quite frankly, jerks. There are big egos at play, but also many brilliant minds. Just remember that you and your doctor both might have strong personalities. There might be insecurities involved, and the constant threat doctors have of malpractice suits. We are the only profession that can be sued for making an informed decision trying to help someone! There are salary cuts and insurance companies for doctors to contend with, but there are also mysterious health conditions that confuse and baffle patients.

It really all boils down to just four things you have to remember:

1. Tell your doctor your symptoms, not your diagnosis of what you think you have.

2. Bring your medical records, but don't interpret them. Let the doctor look at them without your running commentary.

3. Don't tell your doctor too many things at once. Start with the few things that bother you the most.

4. Rather than challenge, test, or lecture your doctor, just ask questions. Maybe you'll get exactly the answers you need.

It might seem to you that you shouldn't have to be responsible for all this special handling with doctors, but doctors also do a lot of special handling when it comes to patients who are scared, angry, or feeling vulnerable. It takes two, so do your part first, and then if the doctor doesn't do his part, find one who does. If you don't feel heard, if you don't feel like he's got it right, if something feels wrong, then you are totally and completely justified in speaking up or moving on. And you can tell him I said so. It is your body, your health, and you need the best health partner/doctor you can find.

Ten Things Your Doctor Should Know About You

Whether you are seeing your doctor for your annual exam or you are in for a particular problem, like heart palpitations or chest pain, there are some basic things your doctor needs to know about you. Be sure you cover these in your visit, or be sure that this information is in your file:

1. Basics of your diet, including how often you eat high-fat or sugary foods, how often you have caffeine, and also how often you eat fruits, vegetables, whole grains, and fish

2. Your waist circumference

3. Your body mass index

4. How often you exercise

5. Your daily stress level: high, moderate, low?

6. Whether and how often you smoke, or whether you were previously a smoker

7. Whether you drink alcohol, and how much

8. Your symptoms. For the sake of your heart, be sure to mention to your primary care doctor and especially to your cardiologist if you have shortness of breath, nausea, jaw pain, back pain, fatigue, chest pain, or any change in your ability to exercise.

9. Your numbers. These should include:
   Total cholesterol numbers, including your LDL, HDL, and triglycerides
   Your hemoglobin A1C
   Your blood pressure
   Your hs-CRP (an inflammation marker)
   Your vitamin D level

10. Whether you have a significant family history of heart disease. This includes any family history of heart attack, stroke, aortic aneurysm, atrial fibrillation or irregular heartbeats, or sudden cardiac death.

What You Want from Your Doctor

Now, let's talk about how doctors should be talking to *you*. There is a thing called patient-centered care, or PCC, that is gaining some momentum in the medical world. Behind it is the revolutionary idea (I use that term sarcastically) that doctors need to listen to patients and include their views and concerns in their care and treatment. This year, the American College of Cardiology Foundation released a health policy statement about patient-centered care that reveals how often doctors don't fully listen to their patients. They are also spearheading efforts to help doctors get better at this. This is an important and necessary innovation in the medical world.

One of the things that stood out for me in the policy statement was this: ". . . upon asking a patient to describe his or her concerns, the clinician interrupted the patient after an average of eighteen seconds; most often, the physician redirected the patient following the first-expressed concern, with subsequent discussion focused solely on that concern."

Now you know this happens because the doctor is trying to construct a differential diagnosis based on that first symptom, but the problem is that you can't get out your whole story in eighteen seconds, not to mention your top five complaints. If you've got one of those eighteen-second doctors, you've got to get to the point, and fast!

The statement also noted: "If patients are given the opportunity to speak without interruption or redirection, they are likely to express three concerns per office visit. Clinicians may be skeptical about allowing a patient to continue until he or she has listed all concerns; however, patients who were allowed to complete their concerns only spoke an average of thirty-two seconds."

In other words, if you are allowed to tell all without interruption, you are likely to spend only thirty-two seconds of your doctor's time. I don't think that's asking too much.

The statement concluded: "The consequences of interrupting initial descriptions of concerns include late-arising concerns and, worse, missed opportunities to gather important information." This is exactly what I was talking about in the last section—extraneous information from you can confuse a diagnosis, but your doctor is equally at fault because interruption and hurrying you along is also likely to cause your doctor to miss important information, or that buried-lede moment when you realize you've left out the most important information of all.

Unfortunately, many doctors have the attitude that what you say isn't what they need to hear. Therefore, they think they need to interrupt you and redirect you. This is likely to happen before you can tell your whole story, robbing you of the opportunity for the best possible diagnosis and cure.

Personally, I don't think I've ever made my point about anything in thirty-two seconds, let alone eighteen seconds, and I'm a doctor (albeit one who might just talk a little too much)!

But now you know how to help. You can tell your story, focus on your most troublesome symptoms, and then let your doctor do his job. You can also seek out a doctor who is interested in your particular problem. For example, if you are interested in prevention, see a doctor who is interested in prevention. If you know you have a specific problem, like diabetes or chronic fatigue syndrome or valve disease, find a doctor with a special interest in that if you can. Ask friends. Ask your primary care doctor. See who's out there. Even ask people on the forums of nonprofit foundations relevant to your condition. You might find out the name of exactly the doctor you need.

Then bring your reports, bring your records, and give them to the doctors, but let your doctor interpret those records, reports, and tests.

If you have a previous diagnosis, say so. If you are looking for a second opinion, say so. If you are having symptoms, say so. If your doctor interrupts you, say, "Just let me finish this thought, please." If you want to be sure you don't forget something important, say, "I do have another concern I want to be sure to mention while I'm here." A good doctor will hear that and make sure you get to express yourself.

Of course, that means you actually have to express yourself. Women often undermine themselves by discounting their own symptoms, and this is a big mistake. Doctors won't necessarily hear that you are scared, or nervous, or afraid to bother anyone. They can't read your mind and they can't feel your symptoms, so they rely on you to give it to them straight. You aren't bothering the doctor, and your symptoms, if you feel them, are not "in your head."

Studies show that one of the main reasons women don't call 911 during a heart attack is that they don't want to be wrong or bother the ambulance drivers or doctors, because maybe they aren't actually having a heart attack. When you give the impression that your symptoms might not be real, your doctor might agree. I've had doctors tell me that their patients seem to "want to be sick," making up symptoms or complaints, but I don't buy this. Not one of my patients has ever wanted to be sick. They might be scared. They might be highly motivated to get to the bottom of their issues, but they aren't trying to manufacture symptoms or get a false diagnosis. Don't make the mistake of sounding like you just want attention but even you doubt your symptoms are valid. Stick to the facts and your doctor will too.

And just so you know, "I don't feel right" is a fact, and you have the right to say it.

It's also important not to discount your own symptoms because you don't have time to be sick. Remember my 37-year-old patient I told you about in Chapter 1? The one who had a massive heart attack and didn't come to see me until three months afterward? When I asked her if she knew what it could be, she said, "I knew it was my heart. I knew it was bad." But she was busy. She didn't have time to be sick, and frankly, she didn't want to know the truth. She ignored her intuition.

It's fine not to make an unnecessary fuss, but if you think you might be having a heart attack, if your heart tells you: *Help!*, if your intuition nudges you and says, "Hey, this is serious," then please listen. The more you delay an intervention, the worse your outcome is going to be. Call the ambulance, go to the hospital, get help when your heart knows you really need it. This is no time to listen to your head.

I believe that with some awareness on both sides, this communication barrier can dissolve. If you are afraid of bothering anybody, that's something for you to work on. If your doctor won't listen to you, that's something for you to speak up about. You deserve to be heard. If a doctor says, "I think it's all in your head," you get to say, "I know my body and this isn't right." You get to explain that you read that some women with the symptoms you have fail to be diagnosed with heart disease, and you don't want to be one of them. I assure you that will get your doctor's attention.

It really comes down to mutual respect, and respect starts with you respecting yourself. Don't dismiss yourself. Don't belittle yourself. And don't ever let any doctor belittle or dismiss *you*. If you are worried about a symptom, say so. If you are interested in holistic treatments in conjunction with your regular care, find a doctor who supports that. If your doctor cuts you off, interrupts you, or isn't giving you the care you really think you need, politely protest. You have the right to quality care, and you have the right to find a different doctor if yours isn't giving you what you need, but first do your best to get the best out of your doctor. Give him a chance, and if he doesn't measure up, then you have every right to go elsewhere.

We are all in this together, doctors and patients. We are all people working our way through this maze of health and disease and wellness. But part of being empowered is to let it start with you, instead of waiting for someone else to do their part first. You just might need some help from your doctor, and now you know exactly how to get it.

This Chapter, by Heart

♥ Your doctor needs to hear your symptoms, not your idea of what you think your diagnosis should be.

♥ The Internet is not a doctor, and it can't diagnose you, although it can be an excellent source of information and you should learn everything you can about your condition from reputable websites.

♥ Your doctor should listen to your story, should not interrupt you, and should not discount your symptoms as "all in your head."

♥ You know about your body. Trust your instincts if you feel that something is wrong, and speak up. Never be afraid to inconvenience your doctor with your genuine problems.

♥ Good doctor-patient communication can start with you, but your doctor must keep up his end of the bargain too. If he doesn't, find a doctor who is particularly interested in your issues, and/or who you feel really hears what you are saying.

PART TWO

What You Should Do

CHAPTER SEVEN

Your Heart Book

You now know a heck of a lot more about your heart and about modern medicine than most people. Congratulations! Now, what are you going to do about it? This is the subject of the next section of this book, and the very first place I want to start is to tell you about my little black book.

No, not *that* kind of little black book. It's a journal I've kept with me ever since the middle of my career, long before I ever became involved with the American Heart Association's Go Red For Women or any of those other national groups. It actually is a little black Moleskine notebook, and it's become a part of my life. Ever since I began practicing medicine, I've been meeting people and hearing stories that made me think, "Women should *know this*. Women should *hear this*. If only all my patients could have heard what this patient just said. If only every woman could hear this story."

So I began to write things down. I wrote down stories of patients. I wrote down things people said that I wanted to remember. I began to write my own story too. And then I began to think: "Everyone should write down their stories. Everyone should record their lives.

My patients should be writing their own stories, so they can look back and read them and begin to realize who they really are." After recommending my patients do this for a few years, I began to call these records of life Heart Books, and this is exactly what this book is for me, the book you are holding in your hands, *Dr. Suzanne Steinbaum's Heart Book*. This is a book about your journey, and my journey too. It's meant to guide you, solely for your own needs, toward a path that will heal and nourish your own heart, and by association, your whole life. So in that spirit, I would like you to start your very own Heart Book. What is your story? And what is your subtitle? Maybe your book will be "Rebecca's Heart Book: A Story of Diet, Exercise, Life, and Love." Or maybe "Jennifer's Heart Book: How to Get Fit, Get Thin, Get Energized, and Get Successful." Figure out what your Heart Book needs to address. What are your greatest heart issues? What are your Heart Throbs? Your passions? Your goals? And where do you want to go next? Make those the heart of your title and fill in your own story. In this chapter, I'll help you get started.

The Heart Book Prescription

When new patients come into my office, I usually begin by having them fill out forms about who they are, their medical and surgical history, medication list, allergies, whether they smoke or drink, their gynecologic history, pregnancy history, what they eat, how much they exercise—the usual doctor stuff, with a few extra lifestyle questions, because that's me.

Then I get to know them. We have a conversation, not just about the symptoms that brought them to the office but about their lives, how they eat, how they exercise, their kids, spouse, work, commute, all of it. I have them fill out a list of stressors, what's going on in their lives, and an anxiety profile and depression scale. I do a physical exam, some blood work, maybe some other tests.

Then I explain what it's going to take to get them feeling better and understanding how to take care of themselves. I always say that we can do this together. And then I say, "Welcome to boot camp." That makes some of them nervous, but still I always say it. I hadn't fully understood why I always say it until recently, when I realized that those words change the mind-set. They understand something when I say "boot camp." They understand that they are embarking on a new stage, a new program for living. I consider it as a welcome into the next stage of health, when they will begin paying attention and taking care of themselves. For some people that really isn't so easy—hence the notion of boot camp. I never want to give anyone false expectations that it is easy. But it is worthwhile—necessary—*crucial*.

All this preliminary work gets them started thinking about where they are and where they need to go, and it's important for me to have all that information. But what's important for the patient is to see their lives in a new way, and to be able to really see the truth about their lives. That will become very clear as they begin to formulate their own Heart Book.

This is when I ask them to start writing down their lives.

I ask them to record their lifestyles. I want to see, and I want *them* to see, exactly what they eat, what they drink, if they exercise, if they had stress and how they managed it, whether they laughed or did things that were fun, how much they slept and if they slept well, and what time of day all these things happened. They can add their details of what mattered to them the most that day, what happened, how they felt that day, if they did something they loved or hated, what they disliked, if they laughed or cried. Sometimes people go all the way with this—they start adding more and more to their books, sharing information like what they enjoyed, what they felt guilty about, how much they connected with others, what in their lives gives them hope or makes them feel calm, and what makes them feel anxious or stressed. I ask them to bring the Heart Book back to me at each appointment, so we can look at it and talk about it together.

I learn a lot from those little black books, computerized diaries, or fancy journals. Many people make their Heart Books part of their days and bring them along wherever they go. Even if your Heart Book is in your smart phone, the information you provide tells an important story.

I'll never forget a patient who came to see me who was having heart palpitations. She was a runner, married with two children, and when she was younger, she used to compete in road races. But after her second child was born, she stopped working and just wasn't feeling well. She didn't have the energy to compete anymore.

We did a lot of tests, and we found that she was experiencing some extra heartbeats. That's when I asked her to start her own Heart Book. Over the course of her treatment, we studied her Heart Book and realized that everything seemed to point to the fact that she had been fairly sedentary and was most likely just out of shape. It is hard to make that diagnosis, especially when someone looks fit and refers to herself as a runner, but when I looked at what she was really doing each day, I saw the truth. It was so simple, but telling a former competitive runner that she was out of shape without being 100 percent sure that it was true . . . well, that was tricky. I decided to do a treadmill test so she could see it for herself. Lo and behold, she was definitely deconditioned. Her heart wasn't working up to capacity because she had stopped exercising, and she was having single early extra beats, easily resolved with drinking more fluids, which she only did after she ran, which she wasn't doing anymore! One thing led to another, and suddenly she wasn't an athlete anymore.

Back to the Heart Book. We also examined what she was eating, and we realized that her nutrition wasn't sustaining her. She simply wasn't eating right. She was on a sugar roller-coaster ride, starting the day with simple sugars and carbohydrates in the morning, crashing by 3:00 p.m., and not having enough energy to play with her children or go for a run later in the day. This is extremely common, but the Heart Book made it perfectly clear that her energy crashes and exhaustion were something she could do something about. After going through her Heart Book, we figured out a better way for her to eat, and then we figured out how she could fit in exercise so she could start working back up to being the athlete she once was. We figured out that in the morning before her husband and children got up, she was doing a lot of things by herself around the house. I suggested that maybe this was the time of day to go out for a run. There was plenty of time for cleaning up toys later, after her children took them all out again after school. Her efforts to be a perfectionist about the clutter in her house were interfering with her efforts to regain her health. I reminded her to stay hydrated and to pay special attention to her water intake on the days she ran.

About three months later, I saw her again, and she was a different person. Her extra beats had stopped. She was exercising regularly. She had changed her diet. She had no more fatigue. And not only did she feel better, she felt whole. She felt like herself again. She was vibrant, vital, and happy, and she told me how much she loved her life. Score one more for the Heart Book!

Now, I could have prescribed a medication to stop those extra palpitations in her chest, but what I wanted for her was more than a prescription. I wanted her to see that she could be the master of her own body, that she could recapture who she really was, and that she could live from the heart. I wanted her to understand that *she* was the one in control of her symptoms. I wanted her to look at her Heart Book and say, "I didn't realize I was doing this! Living like this is not okay with me. This is not working." Because sometimes even if you know, logically, that you aren't living the way you would like to be living, it all becomes so much more clear and manageable when you write it down.

I've seen so many of my patients start a Heart Book and then at some point, maybe a few days or weeks or months after they begin, I see transformation. There is that moment when I see it in a woman's eyes that her life has suddenly become her own again. That moment when she realizes that she can actually do things to feel better. That she has the power over her own life. She understands. And she's empowered. I have seen it in the eyes of the men who really want to make changes in their health and their world too—because all of those men who are part of my practice (almost 40 percent of my patients!) are able to look at themselves in the same critical way, and become equally as accountable for their lifestyle choices. I do have to admit that I sometimes ask the more Heart Book–resistant men to "journal it," and that seems to be a language they like better. I only let them know later that they have created their own Heart Book. Is that sneaky? Of course it's all semantics. Empowerment is never gender specific. It is a universal feeling of mastery, wellness, and sometimes, ultimate happiness.

Now I'm asking you to start a Heart Book of your own.

Your Heart Book

Your Heart Book can be a real book, with a moleskin cover like mine, or a bound book with blank pages, lined or not, or an ordinary spiral-bound notebook or composition book. Or you can keep your Heart Book on your computer, or even in your smart phone. I don't mind where you keep it, but I mind *that* you keep it, because this is the beginning of really knowing exactly who you are. You'll do this by recording your story.

Your Heart Book is yours, so you can fill it up with anything you want, but I would also like you to include information about how you live your life, including what you eat, how much you exercise, and how much you sleep. I'd also like you to write about where you want to be. What do you want from yourself? What do you want from your life right now? What are your goals? Do you want to lose weight? Feel healthier and get in shape? Do you want to feel better about yourself? Sometimes you won't even know what to write down, but as you go through your days, notice the gaps in your life, the voids, or the places where you really want to make changes. Notice the things that you do that make you happy and the times and places that seem to trigger bad habits or self-destructive behavior. Make note of when you put your needs first, and how that makes you feel, and notice when you aren't addressing your own needs at all. Look for patterns. Look for truth.

The more you write, the more you might be inspired to tackle even bigger questions. Are things in your life out of control? Do you want to manage your stress? Do you want to spend more time with the people you love? Do you want to get out of a relationship but you need to take control of your own life and your own health first? Do you want to get into a relationship? Do you want to understand why you have chest pain or do you want to stop the palpitations? Do you want more confidence? Do you want to get pregnant? Do you just want to be present in your life instead of living from your head? Do you want *all of these things*?

Then write it down. There are things in your life that you want to change, that you want to make right. Writing them down makes them real. This is the way to discover what they are, because you might not even be consciously aware of all of them yet. Your Heart Book is your clarifier. It will unveil your habits, your automatic behaviors, the tone you use when you talk to yourself. Once something you've stopped noticing pops back onto your personal radar screen by writing it down, that's when you can seize upon it and realize that eating that bag of popcorn, half a container of ice cream, or that roll of cookies might not have been your healthiest moment.

Many of my patients are completely amazed by what their Heart Books reveal about what they are actually doing. For example, I've had many patients come in with their Heart Books insisting that they have extremely healthy diets and they just don't understand why they aren't losing weight. One of them was living on bagels, muffins, dried fruit, and juice. She thought that was healthy, and she didn't realize that she was eating a diet almost entirely made up of carbohydrates and simple sugars.

Another patient of mine told me that he started every day with a healthy smoothie. He had written down everything he put in it, right there in his Heart Book, for me to see. His smoothie contained low-fat yogurt and nuts and berries, and also flaxseed, and bananas, and apples, and strawberries, and honey or agave. We figured out how many calories were in that smoothie: He was having about 1,200 calories before he even walked out the door! Suddenly it was clear to us both why he wasn't losing weight.

Your Heart Book can reveal how often you *actually* exercise, even if you *intend* to exercise every day. It can reveal why you crash every day at 3:00 p.m. What are you eating for breakfast and lunch? It can also reveal why you are having certain symptoms. I have a patient who was having heart palpitations, and she didn't understand why because she is usually so calm, cool, and collected. Yet every day at 2:00, her palpitations began. So we went through her Heart Book to see what was happening at 2:00 every day. We realized that at 1:30 every day, she had to attend a staff meeting that was over by 2:15. Suddenly she realized how stressful those staff meetings really were to her. She thought she had it under control, and this was just a part of her day. She didn't want to acknowledge that it created anxiety for her, but the body doesn't lie, and neither does the Heart Book, as long as you only write what's true.

So let's get started. If you are one of those people who has never been able to keep a diary, that's okay. Just try this for one week. Just one week, that's all. One week is a snapshot of your life, and it can be incredibly revealing. To help you, I'm going to give you some prompts. The first list includes what I would like for you to record every day, to get a record of your habits and health behaviors. The second list is to help you figure out who you are. Pick one prompt, or more than one if you're feeling like "talking," and write your answer. Don't think about what you're going to write too much. Just start writing. Even if you start with something silly, persevere. If you keep going past the place where you tell yourself you don't know what to say, you'll be amazed at what comes out of your pen or keyboard.

Heart Book Prompts

This first list includes all the things I would like you to record in your Heart Book every day. Consider this a record of *you*. You are your own archivist. This information will not only be illuminating when you look back on it later, but it might also be extremely helpful for your doctor to see if a health issue arises. This list may look long, but it's really not very long once you get used to doing it every day. Let it become a habit, something you do as regularly as brushing your teeth. It's just as important.

I find it interesting that when I start this process for my patients in my office the first couple of days, I get very simple, terse answers, but by day six it usually reads more like a novel of everything that happened in their lives, and why. I love it when this happens! The more you understand that writing will illuminate your triggers and inspirations, the more you will feel empowered to make the changes you know you need to make. And if seven days of writing is enough, then that's enough, but there is some power that comes from writing things down long enough to let your self-exploration and self-realization really evolve. If you can do this for the rest of your life, then more power to you! (And I mean that *literally*.)

In your Heart Book, answer these daily questions:

- What is the date (including the year, because in a few years, you'll want to know)?

- What time did you wake up today?

- How did you sleep?

- How did you feel when you woke up?

- What time did you eat breakfast?

- What did you eat for breakfast?

- How did you feel after breakfast?

- Did you have a midmorning snack? At what time?

- Did you feel like you really needed that snack, or was it more out of habit?

- What time did you have lunch?

- What did you have for lunch?

- How did you feel after eating lunch?

- Did you have a midafternoon snack? At what time?

- Did you feel like you really needed that snack, or was it more out of habit?

- How did you feel midafternoon?

- What time did you eat dinner?

- What did you have for dinner?

- How did you feel after eating dinner?

- How do you feel about what you put into your body today?

- Did you have any pain today? What hurts?

- Did you exercise today? If not, why not?

- How was your energy today? High, low, didn't notice?

- How much water did you drink today?

- Did you laugh today? Did you feel happy? When?

- What was the best thing that happened to you today?

- What was the worst thing that happened to you today?

- Is there anything you did today that you regret or feel guilty about? A few too many cookies? Too many glasses of wine? Harsh words? Something you neglected to do?

- Did you eat a snack after dinner? Did you really want it or was it more out of habit?

- How was your day? Was it a good day, a bad day, a complicated day?

- What time are you going to bed tonight?

- What time did you actually fall asleep? Did you sleep well, or were you restless?

- Did you awake feeling rejuvenated, or were you still tired?

This second list is the "Get to Know Yourself Better" list. Every day, answer one of these questions, or more than one if the spirit moves you. One of my male patients called this the "context." The context is actually the situation under which certain food choices or alcohol choices were made (e.g., a birthday party, you are angry at someone, you had a long, frustrating day at work, it's a night out with your friends). Understanding the context can tell you a lot about why you made the choices you did. These questions are designed to give you a better understanding of your own context, or why you feel the way you do and make the lifestyle choices you make. If any of them seem particularly relevant to your life, you might want to bump them up to the first list and answer them every day.

In your Heart Book, answer one or more of these questions, as you are inspired, or at least think about them. It is an interesting conversation to have with yourself. You can learn a lot.

- Did you do anything today to purposefully reduce your stress level? What was it? How well did it work?

- How do you feel right now at this moment? Do you have a nagging feeling of stress or anxiety that you are trying to ignore? Do you have some physical pain? Do you feel depressed? Write about what might be causing this feeling. Did you eat that half of a chocolate cake because the "context" was that you were stressed over a telephone conversation with your boss?

- How are your hormones? Are you getting PMS? Perimenopausal? Cramps or hot flashes? How well do you think you handle these changing hormonal states?

- Whom do you put first in your life? Whom did you put first today? In what way?

- Do you feel that you give yourself enough attention, or do you feel that you neglect your own needs? Why?

- What are your goals for the next year? Where or how would you like to be one year from today?

- What would you most like to improve about yourself? List five things you could do this week to start moving toward that goal.

- Do you have a ten-year plan? What would you like to accomplish in the next decade?

- How are your personal relationships? Which ones feed you and which ones deplete you?

- If you aren't in a romantic relationship, how do you feel about that? Do you wish you were in one, or are you okay with the way things are?

- If you are in a romantic relationship, are you satisfied with it? What do you like the most about it? What do you like the least about it?

- Do you want to get pregnant? Are you sure? How do you feel about this?

- Are you having health issues? What are they and how do they impact your idea of yourself?

- What life changes do you think would make you feel better?

- Did you feel present in your life today, or distracted? Why?

- Describe yourself as if you were your best friend, really thinking about how others see you and how you project yourself into the world.

- List the things in your life that you feel grateful for.

This list is just a beginning, just a place to start. It is the beginning of awareness, and the beginning of the knowledge that your life is what you make of it, how you choose to view it, and what you choose to do next. Keep it up for as long as you can. If you lapse for a while, start back up. Get to know and love your Heart Book. Commit to it. It's going to help you. It could change your life.

By which I mean it can show you that *you* can change your life.

This Chapter, by Heart

♥ I would like you to start your very own Heart Book, in which you will record the details of your lifestyle choices, like diet and exercise and sleep, as well as the story of your life—how you feel about things, how things affect you, and what you do for yourself.

♥ A Heart Book can help you to uncover why you don't feel your best. It can reveal patterns in your behaviors and choices or help you to see that you aren't eating as well, sleeping as much, or exercising as much as you intend.

♥ Let your Heart Book become something you absolutely love because it helps makes your life better.

CHAPTER EIGHT

Let's Do Some Tests

I t's important to get control of your own information and start recording your life, but it's also important to take that information
and use it to help yourself. This involves your doctor, whether you are
getting your annual checkup or checking into a problem. In order to
help you, your doctor may need to give you some tests. When your
doctor examines you, he can't exactly see your heart, or feel it, or
touch it, or ask it how it's doing. A doctor can't make sweeping statements about exactly what's going on, because of course your heart is
deep inside you, and it's not easily accessible. That's why, when you
have an issue, a pain, a pressure, a palpitation, a thump, a flutter, an
ache, a dizzy spell, or shortness of breath, we have to do tests to figure
out what's going on.

In this chapter, I want to help you understand the tests you are
likely to need, based on your doctor's assessment and the Heart
Throbs you discovered in Chapter 2. Many of the tests I'll talk about
in this chapter are heart-related, although not all of them are. However, the results from all of these tests can help you understand the
areas you need to work on, and the best ways to help your heart, in-

crease your health, and improve your life. Tests and their results aren't always straightforward, and they won't always give your doctor an exact answer, but they can definitely help you to move in the right direction, and sometimes they can give you information you wouldn't have suspected.

This isn't always straightforward. As I explained in Chapter 4, there are four parts to the heart, and all of the symptoms I mentioned on the previous page overlap with each different part. So if you have dizziness, it could be from the muscle, the valve, or the electric system. If you have pain, it could be from the muscle, the valve, the electric system, or the arteries. Depending on your symptoms, and also if your desire is prevention, we start with tests.

Nothing upsets me more than when a patient comes to see me from another doctor, seeking a second opinion, and that person shows me her test results and says, "The doctor said everything is fine. Why do I still feel sick? Why do I still feel like something's wrong?" I start looking at the test and I see things that aren't fine. Maybe the numbers aren't overtly abnormal, but they certainly aren't "fine."

Many times the problems and abnormalities I see are in the lipid profile. When the HDL ("the higher the better") is high, even if the LDL ("the lower the better") is also high, women are told they are "fine" because doctors know (from public health studies) that high HDL is protective. But "fine" is never a way to describe any heart test results, in my opinion. It is a word used to answer the question "How are you?" asked of you by someone you don't know very well. It certainly doesn't give you information.

Sometimes the trouble might be with the blood pressure—that bottom number, the diastolic pressure, is elevated, even if the top number, or systolic pressure, is well within normal range. An elevated systolic pressure is obviously a Heart Throb, but some doctors may overlook a slightly elevated diastolic pressure.

Sometimes I also see so-called fine test results from a stress test that don't look "fine" to me. The results might be technically normal according to parameters established and generally accepted for this test, but when I look at the *patient*, rather than the piece of paper, I see someone who is clearly out of shape, which, as far as the heart is concerned, is not "fine." Or maybe the person had a "normal" result and reached the target heart rate for the test, but she reached it too early in the test, she was short of breath, and her top systolic blood pressure increased to 200 during the test. Test results may be confusing. Patients tend to latch onto them as proof that something is or is not wrong, and doctors do the same thing.

I understand why—tests give us a tangible, researched, and proven way to assess what is really a very complex and multifaceted situation, so it's tempting to give them all the credit. But there are serious problems with overreliance on test results, as well as with ignoring subtle abnormalities in test results. It goes both ways. In this chapter, I want to help you understand what tests can tell you and what they really can't tell you.

For instance, every time you go to the doctor, you get your blood pressure taken. You think, "That's just what they do." But why do they do it? Why is it important? What does it mean? When it comes to really understanding who you are and how to prevent disease in your own body, you need details, even though details aren't the only factor in assessing wellness.

There are many tests for many purposes that look at many aspects of the heart and the other systems in the body. I can't possibly cover them all, but this chapter covers the more common ones you are likely to experience at a visit to your doctor, as well as some heart-specific tests you probably will experience if you or your doctor suspects you might have a heart issue. If you do have a true cardiac issue, you might not find the test your doctor recommends here, and that doesn't mean he's wrong. I'm just giving you a list of the tests I would do that are part of the world of prevention.

Just remember, these tests are only one part of your big picture, but an important part, so let's consider them.

Initial Physical Exam

When you first go to the doctor, perhaps for your annual checkup or maybe because you aren't feeling well, there are some basic things your doctor or the nurse will do: a blood pressure check, a pulse check (which is a check of your heart rate), a general physical exam, a list of questions.

Blood pressure is one of the most basic. You go in, sit on the table or on a chair, you hold out your arm to the level of your heart, a cuff is wrapped around your arm, and the nurse or doctor puts the stethoscope in the crux of your elbow joint and listens with the stethoscope. When the blood pressure cuff releases, your doctor listens for the heart sounds in the artery, which indicate the systolic and diastolic pressure. This test most likely will be repeated every time you visit a doctor's office, because this, along with the pulse and the respiratory rate, or the rate of breathing, are "vital signs," indicating your status as a live person.

When something is amiss with your blood pressure or heart rate, it's a good indication that something is happening inside that shouldn't be happening. It might not be a big, serious thing—it could just be "white coat syndrome," or the tendency to show temporary increased blood pressure and heart rate in the presence of a doctor because doctors make you nervous.

We worry about blood pressure if it is consistently elevated over several readings and over a period of months. We only worry about an elevated heart rate if we think it is a side effect of a medication you are on or if it is associated with symptoms such as dizziness or shortness of breath or passing out. If it is consistently high, indicating poor cardiovascular fitness or an underlying additional problem, such as hyperthyroidism or anemia or even heart failure, we will investigate. A healthy heart shouldn't have to work so hard.

Your doctor will also examine the rest of your cardiovascular system. He will listen to your heart to be sure it sounds normal. (Remember, the doctor can hear certain sounds or murmurs associated with valve disease.) He will listen to your lungs. He will ask you questions about your health and your family history.

Then, if you are having palpitations, chest pain, unusual shoulder or jaw or back pain, or frequent nausea, or if the doctor hears an abnormality in your heart, or if the answers you gave to your doctor's questions and/or your family history suggest you have a lot of Heart Throbs, or if you have any other signs that suggest to a doctor that the problem might be in your heart, your doctor probably will suggest some of the following tests.

EKG or ECG

The next test your doctor is likely to do, especially if you are having some heart symptoms, is an electrocardiogram, commonly referred to as an EKG or ECG. The EKG measures the electrical conduction in your heart. Leads (like little sticky buttons with metal clips) are placed on your chest, arms, and legs. These leads read the electrical impulses in your heart and then the machine interprets them in graphic form, so you get a printout that shows what the heart is doing, including atrium contractions, ventricle contractions, and the pause between the two. The doctor can evaluate the whole conduction system of the heart that makes your heart beat by looking at this printout, which looks a little bit like the printout on a seismograph that would measure earthquake activity or lie detector test results. It's a pretty amazing test—bumps on the graph show when the top part of the heart beats, other spikes reveal when the bottom part of the heart beats. The graph shows not only the heart rate but the rate of speed of that "string of lights" I told you about in Chapter 4 that runs between the top and the bottom parts of the heart.

The EKG can even tell us if there was heart muscle damage from a heart attack, or if the muscle of the heart is strained, thickened, or not functioning optimally. It can tell us about the electrolytes in the body, and whether there is too much or too little potassium and calcium in your system. Sometimes there can be "nonspecific" abnormalities, and these, especially in women, may be a clue to an increased risk of heart disease.

Essentially the EKG is like a map of your heart that your doctor can use to guide you. It doesn't give the details, but it certainly provides an overview of exactly what is going on with the heart in a given moment. The frustrating thing about an EKG is that it is a bit superficial in its data, like a photograph. You can be smiling in one picture and frowning in another—you can guess at someone's mood from a photograph, but you can't know for sure what's really going on. An EKG could at one point be normal and not able to predict or reveal a heart attack that might happen a week from now, so when there are symptoms occurring, often taking serial EKGs, repeating them over a period of time, can give you a better idea as to whether there is anything dynamic or abnormal going on with the heart. Sometimes an EKG can reveal subtleties of an acute coronary syndrome or reveal an irregular heartbeat that looked normal previously. These EKG changes may be the key to a deeper and more complex diagnosis, and can help with efficient and effective diagnosis and treatment.

Echocardiogram

An echocardiogram is an ultrasound of the heart, just like the one doctors use to see the growing fetus during pregnancy, except the probe obviously is moved a little higher up. If there are any abnormalities on the EKG, or there are any heart symptoms or murmurs (those abnormal sounds that your doctor hears when listening to your heart), your doctor might order an echocardiogram to really take a look at what is going on. This ultrasound can see the muscles and valves of the heart, whether the muscles are pumping well or if they are thickened, and whether the valves look normal. It is a moving picture rather than a moment in time, so this gives us more information.

This is the test we use to look at heart function and assess the ejection fraction, or the amount of squeezing of the heart muscle to successfully pump blood. A normal ejection fraction is 55 to 60 percent. Anything below that means that there has been damage to the heart and heart failure can result if the function drops below 40 percent. We can see this on an echocardiogram.

When you get an echocardiogram, you will lie on your left side and get hooked up to the machine with the same kind of leads you would have in an EKG to monitor your heart rate. Then the doctor or a technician puts a clear jelly-like lubricant on a probe with a soft, round, sometimes cold end. (Ultrasound probes and stethoscopes are hard to warm up!) He will place this probe on your chest, and you will both be able to see your heart! Slight pressure might be applied just to push the probe a bit deeper, to see your heart better, but an echocardiogram doesn't hurt. You might be asked to take shallow breaths, or deeper breaths, or to roll more or less to one side or the other, but the whole purpose is to see the heart as clearly and in as much detail as possible. Remember where your heart is located, so you can't get

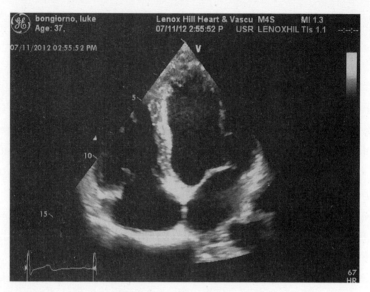

An echocardiogram image of the four chambers of the heart. This is the heart of my physical therapist, Luke Bongiorno.

too shy when your gown might be pulled to the side. That's the only way we can look!

The echocardiogram is able to image all the different parts of the heart, revealing the entire architecture and structure of the heart muscle and walls. It is the "gold standard" for assessing the condition of the heart valves ("gold standard" is how doctors describe the most accepted and proven method to do something), but it can also see all the structures of the heart. We can see the lining of the heart and whether there is any fluid around the heart. Each room or chamber of the heart should be a specific size, with walls of a certain thickness. Measuring these can give us important clues about how the heart is functioning. For example, if the left atrium is larger than it should be, this puts someone at risk for going into atrial fibrillation and may change the treatment plan. One of the first signs of high blood pressure having an effect on the heart is when the left atrium dilates. This is certainly a clue that the blood pressure is not controlled, whether or not the person is on medication. Either way, an aggressive assessment of the blood pressure may be needed, especially if it is "normal" in the office.

But we also get clues for other things. For example, if cholesterol is really high, we might see some calcification on the valves, which is not like the calcium we see in bones but is more in concept like a scarring of the valve. If things get worse, this can lead to the valve being *stenosed*, or having difficulty opening. Ultimately, all those lifestyle choices that lead to the Heart Throbs can take their toll on the valves, the chambers, or the muscle, causing things to not work as optimally as they should. We can see all of this on the echocardiogram.

Holter Monitor, Events Recorders, and Implantable Loop Recorders

Often people having heart palpitations, dizziness, or fainting will not experience these events in the doctor's office, so we don't actually get to hear what's going on with our stethoscopes or see it on an EKG. That's when a doctor might prescribe a Holter monitor or an event recorder.

A Holter monitor is a monitor you wear, usually for twenty-four to forty-eight hours, that keeps a record of what your heart is doing throughout the day and while you sleep. The Holter monitor is hooked up to you using the same type of leads used to connect you to the EKG, with three stickies applied to your chest, which are attached to a small box that you carry on your waistband. Like the EKG, it monitors the heart's electrical activity, so the doctor can see how your heart is beating. It will reveal if the symptoms of palpitations are due to an irregular rhythm, skipped beats, or other irregularities of the electric system.

Strangely enough, I often notice a Murphy's Law kind of situation with the Holter monitor—I will put it on a patient, and during the next twenty-four hours, they feel better than they've ever felt in their lives. Then, as soon as we take it off, they have the worst symptoms they've ever had, with palpitations and a racing heart. When this happens, I sometimes will prescribe an event recorder. This is a slightly different kind of device that you can take on and off and wear for two weeks to a month, as often as possible, in order to pick up an irregular heartbeat to correlate with symptoms. I prescribe an event recorder when an accurate evaluation may require longer than twenty-four hours.

These heart monitors can provide us with useful information, especially when you find your heart symptoms difficult to describe. If you tell your doctor you have a "thingy" going on in your chest, or a "blip," or a "twisting, rushing feeling," or a feeling like your heart is coming out of your chest or is pounding in your throat, to use some common complaints, sometimes the only way to know what that means is by seeing if those symptoms are coming from the rhythm of your heart. That's when a monitor might be recommended.

When there is a symptom of *syncope,* or passing out, the event monitor is often the test of choice. The hope is that you are wearing it the next time an episode happens, and the monitor can pick up whether or not the symptom is related to an irregularity in your heart rhythm.

It's also helpful if you record the time of the symptoms in your Heart Book, so we can compare that to the monitor, correlating symptoms with the heart rhythm. If the symptoms persist, and the monitors don't find anything, then sometimes a small monitor can be implanted under the skin and into the heart, called an *implantable loop recorder,* which gives a continuous monitoring of the electric system. An implantable device can assess the cause of syncope, and the heart rhythm can be monitored over an even longer period of time. This amazing technology sounds like science fiction, but it's very real and can help us figure out what's going on with your heart.

Advanced Lipid Testing

The next test your doctor could possibly do, especially if you have a family history of heart disease or other Heart Throbs, is advanced lipid testing. These are tests beyond the total cholesterol, LDL, HDL, and triglycerides a doctor would typically administer. Advanced lipid testing isn't yet considered standard or mainstream, but I find this information valuable in determining your risk. Lipid tests provide us with information that can help doctors diagnose you, and are also essential for prevention and treatment of the very beginning stages of heart disease.

Lipid test results are among the best predictors of heart disease risk. The tests I recommend include cholesterol (not just HDL and LDL but their various particle sizes, as well as apolipoprotein B, triglycerides, and Lp(a), all of which I told you about in Chapter 2). A lipid test is a simple blood test, best performed after about eight to twelve hours without food in your system. When I know a patient will be having a lipid test, I recommend no food after midnight, and the test at 9:00 a.m. before drinking her morning coffee, although I will check it nonfasting if the patient is on a medication and following a regular healthy diet. Recent guidelines say a nonfasting test may actually be informative, giving insight into a patient's metabolism of carbohydrates, especially if the triglycerides are high. Taking a nonfasting lipid test might be the first clue to a prediabetic condition or a diet that is filled with simple sugars and carbohydrates, so I don't always consider a fasting test to be necessary.

The laboratory can derive a lot of information from that blood sample, giving us a window into your arteries. As I mentioned in Chapter 2, your overall cholesterol number should be less than 200 mg/dl, and your LDL cholesterol should be less than 100 mg/dl. Your HDL goal is greater than 40 mg/dl in men and greater than 50 mg/dl in women, and your triglyceride goal is less than 150 mg/dl. In women, an HDL of 60 mg/dl is the optimum goal and is super protective.

It is clear and obvious that people who have any evidence of plaque in their arteries, or who have had a heart attack, should have an LDL number less than 70 mg/dl (preferably closer to 50), and in those with diabetes or other Heart Throbs, that number should definitely be less than 100.

However, that doesn't mean that if your LDL number is 130 mg/dl, you are doomed. It just means you have to work on your diet and exercise to get it lower. If it is greater than 160 mg/dl, medication might be the next step. The goal for LDL is very dependent on your level of wellness and whether you have other Heart Throbs. If you are super-healthy, exercise, and have a great diet and a high HDL, an LDL above 130 mg/dl is considered perfectly acceptable by the standard guidelines. I look at it a bit differently. I see it as a place to make a change, before the HDL drops and the LDL rises, as it often does with aging. This leads me to my initial recommendation, which is to make it a goal to get the LDL less than 100 mg/dl, no matter what your risk is. Many times, this can be achieved through lifestyle modification. If not, we may need medications.

Statins are a class of medication used to lower LDL cholesterol. There are different types that have different properties based on their strength and the duration of their action, but all of them offer benefits beyond lowering "bad" cholesterol. Remember the endothelium? The plaque that develops inside the endothelium is filled with cholesterol and inflammatory cells, and it is covered with a fibrous cap. Statins stabilize this plaque and thicken the fibrous cap so it does not rupture by decreasing inflammation. Remember, a plaque rupture means a piece breaks off, causing platelets to seal up the tear, blocking blood flow to the muscle of the heart, which then leads to a heart attack. Plaque rupture is what most often leads to heart attacks, and the statin is able to turn an unstable plaque into a stable plaque. This medication is the most potent anti-inflammatory for plaque, which is critical in preventing acute coronary syndromes and heart attacks, as we discussed in Chapter 4.

Statins can be a valuable medication for those at risk, but their use *does not* preclude diet and exercise as highly effective managers of a high LDL. However, if you do have plaque that is unstable, with inflammation (see the section on inflammation later in this chapter), statins are proven to be the most protective intervention.

The HDL is the good stuff. It protects the arteries by shuttling out the LDL particles (as I explained in Chapter 2). HDL stays elevated with estrogen, so most premenopausal women have high HDL levels, which is one of the reasons women were always considered to be at low risk for heart disease. HDL also stays elevated with a healthy diet and regular exercise, and in fact, exercise is the most effective lifestyle practice that can increase the HDL. In an analysis of fifty-two exercise trials, HDL went up as much as 4.6 percent over twelve weeks.

When HDL is less than 50 mg/dl in women, and 40 mg/dl in men, the risk of heart disease increases. In fact, women who have low HDL may be at a greater risk of heart disease than men with low HDL. According to the Framingham Heart Study, there is a fivefold increase in the predictive risk of heart disease with a low HDL, and for every 1 mg/dl drop in HDL, there is a 2 to 3 percent increased risk in men and a 3 to 4 percent increased risk in women. With an HDL level below 40 mg/dl, a statin should be considered as part of a preventive strategy. When we see young people with premature onset of heart disease, a low HDL is often the culprit. Many trials have looked at medications to raise the HDL, and so far we are waiting for that magic pill. Niacin in a long-acting form had been the treatment of choice, but for people who have low HDL due to their high triglycerides, niacin could increase the risk of stroke, and should not be used. But of course you might be able to guess my prescription to raise HDL: Get on the treadmill, or do something to get your heart rate up.

If you are a woman, your estrogen will eventually decrease, so you have to exercise to keep your HDL elevated.

The next part of the lipid panel is the apolipoprotein B, which directly correlates to the more dangerous, small, dense particles of LDL cholesterol. In women, this number might be more predictive of heart disease than the LDL alone. The goal is to have a test result number less than 80 mg/dl (depending on the particular lab). This is one of those numbers that can be lowered with diet and exercise, but if it is really high, then statins would be the drug of choice.

Heart Beats

If you don't have access to an apolipoprotein-B test, or your doctor doesn't think it is necessary, you can calculate your non-HDL cholesterol on your own. Take your total cholesterol minus your HDL cholesterol. According to the National Cholesterol Education Panel III, this value gives an understanding of how much of the lipid panel is plaque forming. The goal is a non-HDL of less than 130 mg/dl, and if it is greater than 160 mg/dl, then it is very high. Between 139 and 159 mg/dl is borderline, and all measures of diet and exercise should be part of the aggressive management strategy. If these aren't enough, medication is indicated.

Triglycerides, another component of cholesterol, are directly related to the food you eat. Triglycerides should be less than 150 mg/dl. Triglycerides are often associated with a diet heavy in carbohydrates and sugars, and a high number is a sign that you are headed toward a prediabetic or diabetic condition, as high triglycerides are often associated with insulin resistance.

In this scenario, simply getting the triglycerides down will raise the HDL. If the triglycerides are greater than 200 mg/dl, and the HDL is lower than 40 mg/dl, the recommendation is to take a fenofibrate, which is a medication to treat this issue. Omega-3 or an EPA/DHA supplement in the form of fish oil or krill oil is also a good idea. You can take up to 4 grams a day. Brands with a higher ratio of EPA to DHA are the most effective.

Lipoprotein (a), also called Lp(a), is a protein that is attached to the LDL particles. As I mentioned in Chapter 2, high levels of Lp(a) are inherited and not based on or corrected by lifestyle, and are associated with an increased risk of heart disease and stroke. I remember starting my fellowship and seeing a young, physically fit 32-year-old man with a perfect cholesterol panel and great diet being wheeled into the emergency room with a heart attack. No one could understand why he had a heart attack. This was early in the field of prevention, but we checked for this marker and found it was elevated. If you have a family history of heart disease, this might be one to check, because even if you are doing all the right things, this marker will increase your risk independently. The only treatment for this is niacin in a long-acting form, although we still don't have the data to prove that niacin works to prevent heart attacks. Some studies say it does, and others suggest it doesn't.

Heart Beats

A recent study published in August 2012 suggested that blood type might influence coronary heart disease risk. In the study, people with AB blood type (the rarest type, found in only 7 percent of the U.S. population) had a 23 percent increased risk of heart disease compared to those with the most common blood type, type O (found in about 43 percent of the U.S. population). Those with type B blood had an 11 percent increased risk, and those with type A had a 5 percent increased risk compared to those with type O. The results were based on two large studies, including the Nurses' Health Study, which included 62,073 women. We don't know for sure that this result is unique to women, but it definitely was apparent in women. Study participants were between the ages of 30 and 75 and were followed for twenty years or more.

There is evidence that people with type A blood tend to have higher levels of LDL cholesterol, and that type AB may be linked to inflammation. There is also evidence to suggest that people with type O have healthier endothelium and less clotting.

This is just one example of new research that hasn't yet been integrated into clinical care, let alone fully understood, but it's interesting nevertheless. It certainly wouldn't hurt those with blood type A to limit fat intake, and for those with blood type AB to monitor inflammation.

High-Sensitivity C-Reactive Protein

If you are at risk for heart disease, another important test for inflammation is a blood test called the high-sensitivity C-reactive protein test. In 2008, a study was published in the *New England Journal of Medicine* called the JUPITER Trial. This trial was pivotal in giving us an understanding that risk is not just about LDL cholesterol but also about what is going on inside the plaque that is forming within the lining of that artery. It showed us that with inflammation, there is an increased risk of heart disease, which doesn't surprise us now, because we learned that plaques filled with cholesterol and inflammatory cells are more likely to rupture and cause a heart attack than stable plaque.

The test for inflammation is a blood test, and the most telling marker is the presence of hs-C-reactive protein, also called high-sensitivity CRP. The trigger to release CRP into the bloodstream comes from the presence of macrophages (part of the immune response to plaque), or when there is an increase in fat cells. This is common in people with an increased waist circumference, which independently increases cardiovascular risk. Other markers, such as an Lp-PLA2, are also linked to inflammation, and some studies have shown that when this is elevated along with CRP, the risk for heart attack increases. You are at a low risk of developing cardiovascular disease due to inflammation if your hs-CRP level is lower than 1.0 mg/L. You are at average risk if your levels are between 1.0 and 3.0 mg/L, and high risk if your level is above 3.0 mg/L.

When the risk of heart disease is borderline or intermediate, meaning you have one or two risk factors, then sometimes CRP can tip the scale. If the hs-CRP is elevated, then doctors are more likely to treat you more aggressively in order to prevent heart disease. The first step is to change your diet and increase your exercise, because both these lifestyle changes can decrease inflammation. As your risk increases with an elevated CRP, your doctor might also prescribe an aspirin regimen and/or other medications to lower your cholesterol and blood pressure.

Interestingly, CRP can go up with an increase in belly fat, so if you have a bit of a paunch, are eating too many cookies in front of the TV, and have an elevated CRP, maybe the first step is to lose the belly fat. The CRP just might come down on its own.

Hemoglobin A1C

As long as you are giving away all this blood, you might as well give some for the hemoglobin A1C test, also called the HBA1C in doctor lingo. Unlike some tests, which are influenced by what you ate that day or the day before, this test takes a longer view. It is a useful test to screen for diabetes and also to make sure that if you do have diabetes, you've got it under control.

Even though a fasting blood sugar can give us a clue whether or not you have prediabetes or elevated sugars, this test allows us to see what your blood sugar has been over a period of time, not just the past day when you were on your best behavior because you knew you were going to be taking a blood test.

Ideally, your HBA1C should be below 5.7. If it is between 5.7 and 6.0 and you were in my office, you and I would have a long and serious discussion about your food intake. If it was greater than 6.0 to 6.4 percent, then I would prescribe a no-sugar boot camp, a complete analysis of your diet, a fierce exercise plan, and possibly even medication. Greater than 6.5 percent is the diabetic range, and we will implement a new diet, exercise, and medication until you get your sugars under control on your own. The goal for the HBA1C if you have diabetes is less than 7 percent.

If you are strict with yourself, your sugars will come down quickly. One of the easiest and fastest ways to do this is to stop drinking any sugar-sweetened beverages, then recheck in three months. This can make a huge difference, and you'll see that you can actually prevent or reverse diabetes in yourself! Now, that's empowering.

ApoE

The ApoE test is another blood test. It is a genetic test that can tell us how people metabolize certain foods, like fats and carbohydrates. This test helps determine the activity of the enzymes that shuttle the cholesterol through the body and the enzymes involved in breaking down the fats we eat. This is extraordinarily helpful to understand how much these foods play a role in the cholesterol panel and can help guide dietary changes, giving us an understanding of what your risk of heart disease is, based on the genes you inherited and how that relates to the food you eat.

I know that at this point, you are an expert in understanding that what you eat can affect your heart, but each individual may possess a gene that doesn't allow the body to process foods without having them lead to elevated LDLs or exorbitantly high triglycerides. This is why not all people do well on the same diets. Some thrive on a very low-fat diet. Others require more fat and can't handle simple carbohydrates and sugars.

In Chapter 2, I explained that there are three of these ApoE genes: ApoE2, ApoE3, and ApoE4. Everybody has two, and you can get them in any variation. Which ones you have can tell us a lot about your individual body's metabolism. The majority of people, about 60 percent, have two ApoE3 genes.

The ApoE4 gene is found in about 25 percent of the population and is associated with an increased risk of heart disease. When someone has an E4 isoform of the ApoE, fats cannot be broken down and absorbed, and the LDL cholesterol skyrockets, leading to plaque formation. Those people who have E4 don't break down LDL as efficiently, and the receptors that essentially sweep up the LDL are suppressed, so those people who have E3/E4, or especially E4/E4, are at greatest risk for developing heart disease because of the difficulties managing fats. The ApoE4 is also associated with Alzheimer's disease, but it is not specifically diagnostic of the disease, nor does it mean that you are going to get it.

If you carry this genotype, then it is imperative to be on a very low-fat diet, with less than 7 percent of your calories from saturated fats. The truth is that if you carry this gene, you are the type of person that should be on a vegetarian or vegan diet. Medications alone are not beneficial, and both medication and dietary changes are usually needed.

The ApoE2 genotype is associated with lower LDL levels but elevated triglycerides. This is a metabolic problem seen in the genetic disorder type III dysbetalipoproteinemia, which is a rare inherited disorder causing fatty yellowish deposits on the skin and increased triglycerides, along with early-onset atherosclerosis. If you have an ApoE2 gene, it doesn't mean that you have this rare disorder, but it does mean that you have difficulty metabolizing carbohydrates. Oftentimes with this genotype, there is an associated prediabetes or diabetes, along with overweight or obesity. The best solution is changing the diet to a very low-carb diet, and everything will resolve, including the high triglycerides.

The ApoE test might sound really interesting to you, but you might have trouble getting it because doctors don't normally prescribe this test and the FDA has not recommended it as a test that should be used for everyone. In my office, however, I find that for people who are having cholesterol issues or problems with LDL and triglycerides, it is helpful to get this information to figure out the best individualized diet plan. Many times when we find out the results, my patients will say something like "I had a feeling I had that problem."

I recommend you take a guess about your own metabolism. How do you feel after you eat fats or carbohydrates? If either of those affect you negatively, cut them out of your diet and see if you feel better.

Stress Test

A stress test is the traditional test used to detect blockages in the arteries. Sometimes when I suggest doing a stress test, my patients say something like "Every day of my life is a stress test!" That might be true, but this is a different kind of stress. It doesn't actually measure your mental stress. It measures your ability to exercise.

Usually doctors will conduct a stress test if you have been experiencing chest pain or shortness of breath. The stress test can evaluate whether your symptoms are due to blockages in your arteries. It can also detect what is happening with your electrical system and your blood pressure during exercise. The concept of the stress test is one of supply and demand. When the heart is under the stress of exercise, the demand for oxygen goes up. If blockages in your arteries are 70 percent or greater, then the supply of oxygen goes down under the stress of exercise. That mismatch is what leads to symptoms of angina or heart pain, and sometimes shortness of breath, nausea, back pain, jaw pain, sweating, or whichever brand of angina you tend to get, and is the reason that your stress test would be considered "abnormal." The frustrating thing is that this so-called gold standard for testing arterial blockages only tells us if the blockages are greater than 70 percent. It doesn't tell us if they are 30 percent or 50 percent, which are the most likely culprits leading to a heart attack because they are the most likely to rupture. If your stress test is "normal," it doesn't mean you can't have a heart attack, so I never rely on this test alone to detect arterial blockages or heart attack risk.

There are many different kinds of machines that give stress tests, the most common being the arm ergometer or the treadmill. Sometimes medication is used in the vein to simulate the heart's response to exercise. This is done if someone can't walk (for instance, they might have a broken leg), or for someone who has specific abnormalities on an EKG.

When you take a stress test, in most cases you will walk on a treadmill that gets progressively faster and steeper. You are hooked up to an EKG machine while you are on the treadmill, in order to monitor your heart rate and to look for abnormal heart rhythms associated with your increasing exercise effort. Your blood pressure is also taken intermittently throughout the test to determine your body's response to exercise. The "stress" in this situation is exercise.

As the treadmill gradually goes faster and the incline gets steeper, the doctor tracks how long it takes you to get to your target heart rate. The intensity of each stage on the treadmill is measured in METs, which stands for metabolic equivalent of task. METs are a somewhat arbitrary way of assessing how much oxygen is required for that particular level of effort on the treadmill. One MET is the amount of oxygen required at rest. If you achieve your target heart rate in the first stage of the stress test, at a low level of METs for your age, then let's face it, you are out of shape. Your heart rate shouldn't go up that quickly. There is usually a standard protocol, with each stage increasing in speed and incline (unless you are using an arm bike, in which case the resistance goes up), and a point at which you are expected to reach your target heart rate. If it takes a long time to reach your target heart rate, then you are officially in great shape.

Your performance on the treadmill is determined by the amount of time you exercise, EKG changes, and symptoms. Using the three variables, we can figure out your risk of heart disease. In fact, if you do fabulously well, then we know you have a pretty good chance of glowing health for about the next four years and are very unlikely to have a heart attack (if, of course, you keep all the other Heart Throbs in check).

Sometimes your doctor will do an imaging procedure before and after the stress test, like an echocardiogram, or use a nuclear camera, which images a radioisotope that is injected into a vein. This radioisotope grabs onto red blood cells and the camera shows where those red blood cells go. If there is a blockage, then there will be less radioisotope in that area during exercise. These imaging procedures allow your doctor to see your heart at rest, and then again after exercise. If the supply of oxygen from one artery is decreased, then that wall of the heart to which that particular artery supplies oxygen will not receive the blood tagged with the radioisotope and will not show up on the stress test images. We can actually see this obvious mismatch between "rest" and "stress" (the exercise state). This can help your doctor clarify whether you will need an angiogram or further evaluation.

An echocardiogram, along with a stress test, can also look for blockages in the arteries, as well as assess the function of the heart valves and determine the proper timing for surgery if the valves are too tight or too leaky. It can also be used to assess the effectiveness of a prior treatment, like a stent or medication.

However, I believe the greatest part of a stress test is that it can assess your heart's true cardiac vitality. Seeing your heart under working conditions demonstrates how vital it is and how physically fit you are. This is the primary reason I use a stress test: to determine your fitness. If you aren't fit, regular exercise is the prescription. I say it to all my patients, and I've said it to you before, but I'll say it again: Exercise is the best medication. (I talk more about exercise and stress tests in Chapter 10.)

Calcium Score

The coronary artery calcium score is a controversial test. In the cardiology world, there is a large school of thought that believes it is unnecessary and does not help provide any additional information beyond the tests we already use. Before you ask your doctor for this test, it might help you to know a little bit more about it.

Essentially, a calcium score is a CT scan. You lie down on a table, hold your breath, and snap! An X-ray type of machine takes a picture of your heart. When your doctor evaluates the images, he can see calcium within the arteries. Remember when I told you that plaque develops a fibrous cap that gets thicker and more stable as it matures? This cap has calcium in it, and the calcium is counted and assigned a score. I think of this test as the equivalent of a mammogram, but for the heart, because it is a picture that is used as a screening tool that gives us an overall analysis but doesn't necessarily catch everything.

A trial called the Multi-Ethnic Study of Atherosclerosis (MESA) shows that calcium in the arteries is associated with an increased risk of heart disease. Your individual calcium score is compared against what's appropriate for your age group. If you are at a level above the 75th percentile for your age, your risk is significantly higher than normal. The problem with the calcium score test is that it doesn't show goopy, immature "baby plaque" (the cardiology world calls this "low attenuation plaque," which is more unstable) that is not calcified yet, so your score might not give an accurate picture of the state of your plaque. Not everyone needs this test. If all your Heart Throbs are in check and other basic test results look fine, then there is no reason for it. But if you have a strong family history of heart disease or if some of your other cholesterol markers or genetic markers are elevated, or you have multiple other Heart Throbs, then this test might be helpful in determining if in fact you are at risk and need aggressive prevention, which might include medication, like taking an aspirin a day.

Studies have shown that people who are aware that they have a high coronary artery calcium score are more compliant in taking their medication as well, so there is something to be said for doing the test and communicating the results when they show something significant. The empowering thing is that if you have a calcium score of 0 and an excellent stress test, your risk of heart disease for the next four years is very low.

Carotid Doppler

Carotid dopplers use ultrasound to look at the carotid arteries. Using the same technology as the echocardiogram, this ultrasound probe (with the same clear jelly) is applied to your neck while you lie on a table, neck turned to either side, so the arteries are accessible to the ultrasound. This is similar to the echocardiogram, but it looks at the arteries in your neck to assess something called the carotid intima-media thickness, or CIMT. The test measures the thickness of the carotid artery to assess the development of plaque. As a test, the progression of thickness in the carotid artery can be extrapolated to the heart, as all the arteries are lined with that same endothelium, and a problem in one set of arteries means that there might be a problem in another set—in this case, the heart arteries. By evaluating and tracking the CIMT, doctors might make an assumption that there is plaque buildup throughout the arteries of the heart. If the progression of growth is greater than 0.1 mm per year, then aggressive preventative treatment becomes necessary.

As with the calcium score, those who are above the 75th percentile for their age or those with a thickness exceeding 1.5 mm are considered at high risk for heart disease. In a study called the Framingham Offspring Study cohort, the CIMT was added to the traditional Framingham risk analysis, and more effectively predicted who was at risk for heart disease than predictions based on the standard risk markers alone. This test can be used the same way as the calcium score to determine who is making too much plaque for their age.

CT Scan Angiogram

The CT angiogram is a CT scan that looks at your arteries. You lie on a table and dye is injected into your vein through a catheter. (If you are allergic to shellfish, let your doctor know because you might have a reaction to the contrast dye that is typically used for this test.) A big camera takes a picture of your heart in tiny slices. The computer then reconfigures the heart into a three-dimensional view. Very high-tech and incredibly amazing to look at!

There has been some controversy about this test, and it is definitely not recommended as a screening test because of the radiation involved. Any test that requires radiation must be administered only when necessary, because the benefit must outweigh the risk of radiation exposure.

I often use this test to make a final assessment in many of my patients who persistently have symptoms but who have normal stress tests. The CT angiogram is 98 percent sensitive in diagnosing obstructive heart disease compared to the stress test, which is 69 percent sensitive. (This sensitivity percentage is based on how likely the test is to show an abnormality when the patient is actually sick.) The CT angiogram can also tell if a plaque is calcified and stable, or if it has *low attenuation,* meaning it is not stable. Sometimes the CTA really can determine if the symptoms are coming from the heart or not in someone who continues to have symptoms but who has normal results on all other tests. Not every hospital has the machine to do this test, but if you have access to one, talk to your doctor about whether or not this test makes sense for you.

Catheterization or Angiogram

The coronary angiogram is absolutely the most definitive test for looking inside the arteries. However, it is an invasive test, so you will have to go into the hospital for this one. It is done in a sterile environment, so get ready to get gowned and washed down with disinfectant. A small puncture is made in the femoral artery in the groin or in the radial artery in the wrist, and a catheter is fed right to the top part of the heart, through the internal network of arteries that branch off the aorta. Dye is injected through that catheter, and through a fluoroscopy imaging, we can then see the arteries on a TV screen. By looking at the image, we can see blockages that might require a stent, which we can actually place during this procedure if necessary.

Heart Beats

A stent is a tiny mesh metal straw placed inside an artery to hold it open in the area where there is a blockage. There are many kinds of stents. Some are bare metal and others are "drug eluting," which means they are coated with a medication to prevent the stent from closing up. The reality is that ultimately, these stents are not a cure. They are simply a bandage to help the artery work better. They do not prevent heart attacks and death, but when someone is having a heart attack, this is a life-saving procedure that allows the heart muscle to get oxygen.

During the catheterization, your doctor can also do an intravascular ultrasound, which can measure the inside of the artery and look closely at the condition of the plaque inside it to determine its composition (hardened or "goopy") and whether it is stable or vulnerable. This is important, because we now know we cannot just focus on plaque prevention. We also need to focus on stabilizing existent plaque and decreasing the inflammation that leads to rupture. This test can help clarify what kind of preventive actions are necessary, and can also look at the diffuse plaque women tend to get, which is different from the more obvious obstructions men tend to get. Sometimes the plaque women get is hard to see, and the IVUS will help detect it.

There are many other tests your doctor might suggest based on your symptoms; this is just an overview of some of the major heart-related tests that are relevant to your heart health, heart care, and wellness. It might seem like an intimidating list, but my take-home message for this chapter is that there are many ways to assess what might be wrong with your heart. Please don't be afraid of tests! No test is perfect, but cardiology and technology have come a very long way in helping doctors take care of you. Tests can give you information, and information is power. And if a test does reveal a problem, the sooner you find it, the better off you will be. You will *know*, and that means you can control what you do next, including controlling the many lifestyle factors that directly affect how healthy your heart will be tomorrow.

This Chapter, by Heart

There are many tests doctors might do to assess your general health and specifically your heart health, or to get to the bottom of heart symptoms. The tests I am most likely to recommend in my cardiology practice are:

- ♥ General physical exam, including blood pressure and heart rate

- ♥ EKG

- ♥ Echocardiogram

- ♥ Holter monitor

- ♥ Event recorder

- ♥ Advanced lipid testing, including LDL, HDL, apolipoprotein B, triglycerides, and Lp(a)

- ♥ hs-CRP

- ♥ Hemoglobin A1C

- ♥ ApoE

- ♥ Stress test

- ♥ Coronary artery calcium score

- ♥ Carotid doppler

- ♥ CT scan angiogram

- ♥ Catheterization or angiogram

CHAPTER NINE

Your Dietary Action Plan

Eating and moving are such instinctual actions that you would think they would be the simplest parts of our lives to navigate. Eating food and walking around the block are much easier than getting a job or maintaining a relationship or raising children, don't you think? Shouldn't it be a simple matter of logic, of math, of checks and balances? Animals eat and exercise without messing it up, and the only fat animals I've ever seen are the ones who are fed by humans.

Yet eating and exercise have become two of our biggest human challenges. Losing weight seems like it should be a matter of a very basic equation: calories in versus calories burned. Manipulate that ratio and lose or gain weight. It's science. It's not complicated. So what's wrong with us? Why are we so sick, overweight, tired, frustrated, and completely unable to make change happen in our lives? Why is it so hard to eat and exercise and live in a way that will keep us slim, strong, and heart-healthy?

I believe the reason humans have so much trouble practicing a healthy lifestyle is simple. When we plan and try to execute our diets and workout routines, and especially when we think about how our bodies should look, we are living from our heads. We are *deciding* how to get healthy instead of *feeling* how to be healthy. As soon as you've got restrictions on what you can eat, you begin to think about food all the time, even when you're not hungry. We don't eat when we're hungry and we eat when we're not hungry, and we obsess and torture ourselves and deprive ourselves and generally feel miserable.

This is often how it goes. First, you notice something about yourself you don't like—big thighs or a chunky butt or cellulite or a muffin top, or maybe it's a lack of muscle tone or just low energy and a blah feeling. Next, you feel guilty that you've let yourself go so drastically (even when it's not drastic). Clearly, something must be done. So you make a very sensible plan for fixing your obvious personal failings. Maybe you find it in a book, or on the Internet, or you decide to do a diet a friend suggested. You get excited. You get hopeful.

You wake up ready to start! You go to the book or the chart or the list and see what you are allowed to eat for breakfast. As soon as breakfast is done, you start thinking about what you are allowed to eat for lunch. Maybe you'll even enter it into your calorie counter app ahead of time, in anticipation.

You watch the clock, waiting for the next time you are allowed to eat. You portion out your meals with measuring cups and spoons. You arrange your food so it looks attractive, or you eat your boring diet food and wish it looked better. When you finally get to eat, you feel both virtuous and dissatisfied. It wasn't enough, or it didn't taste good, or it wasn't the food you really felt like eating. But at least you stuck to the plan!

Then the gnawing begins at the edges of your consciousness and you start thinking about those potato chips or cookies in the pantry or the vending machine, or the candy bowl at the office, or a big plate of crisp nachos or cheese fries or pizza. You can't get images of those forbidden foods out of your mind. You intellectualize: You must be hungry. You should eat a healthy snack. So you have a bowl of whole-grain cereal with skim milk or a fruit smoothie or some yogurt, and yet the candy bowl is taunting you, teasing you in the recesses of your mind, until eventually you can't stop *thinking* about it.

Then life happens. You get invited out to dinner or to a friend's house. Everyone at work goes out for lunch. Or you forget to go to the store. Suddenly you panic. Are you on the first week of this new diet or the second week? Which part of the week, and which foods are allowed when? Can you go out to eat? Oh no, you forgot to bring your diet book with you! Is this food on the list? *If I eat this, will I ruin everything? But I really want to eat this! Why can't I just relax and have fun?* Then you start feeling sorry for yourself, neglected and famished and miserable from the denial and intense discipline your new diet demands of you. It's all so unfair!

Then fun wins out. You eat, and eat, and eat. It's all ruined. You're shocked. You're disillusioned. You conclude that you are weak or that the plan was wrong and you need a different one. Or you give up and decide to go back to your old habits. You obviously fail at dieting, so you don't even think about making healthy choices anymore. And then you notice something about yourself you don't like—were your upper arms this jiggly before? And the whole ridiculous process begins again.

Ladies, this is no way to live. This is no way to eat. And, I would argue, this is no way to take care of your heart. The stress alone from obsessing about dieting is damaging, not to mention the binge that is likely to follow your days or weeks of so-called restraint, and the strain on your body from constantly gaining and losing and regaining weight.

I'd like you to count how many diet books you have. How many diets have you tried? How many successes have you celebrated, how many failures have you suffered, how many times have you said to yourself, "I've got to stop eating like this! I've got to get back to the gym! I've got to start a new plan!"

And how many times have you given up?

When you are on a diet, your whole body aches with *want*. You *want* that cookie-dough ice cream, those French fries, that pasta, that Cosmopolitan, and then you're sunk. You've blown it. So you keep eating to fill that hole that seems to grow ever wider and deeper, until you feel hopeless at the thought of ever feeling satisfied again.

I know what this feels like because I've been there myself. But I also know that you don't have to live like that anymore. Let's be done with all that torture, shall we? Let's be done with it, with the calm reassurance that giving up dieting will *not* doom you to obesity. In fact, I happen to know that it will do just the opposite: It will finally grant you glowing heart health *and* the graceful figure that is the healthy heart's happy by-product.

What You Really Want

As a cardiologist, I see this vicious dieting cycle playing itself out time and time again because the inevitable effects of overeating, or eating too much sugar and saturated fat, especially coupled with guilt and anxiety, often lead to heart disease. That's when people come to see me—when they are at the end of their proverbial rope. I wish they would come to me before things got so desperate that they feared for their heart health. I want you to start making changes *before* you have to make an appointment with a cardiologist, so let's get right to work. You've got no more time to lose—and enough with the self-torture too!

Let's start with food. I believe most of the time, when people crave foods they know aren't good for them, especially when they are well fed and not physically hungry, it is because they want *something*.

They only *think* they want food. The mind justifies what the body is doing, making spurious connections like "If you eat cake, you will feel loved," or "If you lie on the couch staring at the TV, you will feel rested."

But the mind is wrong! It gets confused. It draws false conclusions and relies on faulty logic. Not always, of course, but often, especially where the body is concerned. The body is smart and it knows how to trick the mind into justifying what's the easiest and most comfortable option in the moment. The body doesn't look to its future, and so the mind complies with the body's demands. The truth lies somewhere else, somewhere in the middle. Your heart knows what you really need, even as the mind plays tricks on itself to justify the body's comfortable habits. This is why an intellectual approach to figuring out what you *really* want is nearly impossible. You have to feel it.

The only way to transcend the body's whiny demands and the mind's hamster-wheel obsessions is to get right in the center of your being and *listen*. This is how you live from the heart. Before any diet or exercise plan will work, you absolutely have to feel what you really want. Only then will you have the passion and motivation to do the work to get it.

Ask yourself the following questions, and don't think about them. Just answer directly, based on your feeling. Feel the answers as they come from your heart, rather than your brain. Write them down if you want to be sure you remember, although you don't have to. Many of these questions have yes or no answers, and those answers will change as you change. Answer the questions according to how you feel in your current state, right this minute:

- Do you want more affection?
- Do you want more attention?
- Do you want more energy?
- Do you want more sensual pleasure?

- Do you want more appreciation for what you do?
- Do you want to feel attractive?
- Do you want to feel calm?
- Do you want to be stimulated?
- Do you want adventure?
- Do you want to be freed from too many responsibilities?
- Do you just want some peace and quiet?

Every single one of these questions is much more likely to lead you to helpful and fulfilling answers than the question "What can I eat right now?" The answers to these questions are not inside the refrigerator. They are inside *you*. The answers are in your heart, and you will find them when you learn to live by the heart. The mind is ever-changing, but the heart knows what it really wants, and I can tell you right now that your heart does not want a cheeseburger, a pound of pasta, a candy bar, or a Cosmopolitan. What's the momentary experience of gulping down a cheeseburger when you put it up against "more affection" or "peace and quiet" or "adventure" as a goal for your day?

Food is a tool, not a goal. Food can optimize our bodies and minds so we can best get the things we want. That's not to say you can't enjoy your food. Of course you can, and you should. Food is one of life's great pleasures, but it's not an end in itself. It's like a pretty dress or a power tie, like beautiful weather or a smile from someone on the street. It can enhance your life, but it's not your ultimate achievement.

This is a hard leap to make, especially when we get too attached to food or we use it in place of emotional fulfillment, which is very common. But what do we do to fix the problem? Most of the people I know think it to death! We are so attached to a life lived in the brain. For some strange reason, we can't stop running around in those mental circles.

However, this is the most important thing to understand if you are going to heal your heart: You have to start living from your center, not from your intellect. The mind has its place and its purpose, but when thinking and intellectualizing are not working for you when it comes to your health, then it's time to try something different.

Learning What to Do

In my experience, people really don't know how to get the things they want, and that's okay. You may come to the realization that you want more love, not more cheesecake, but how do you get it? The cheesecake might seem a lot easier to acquire, although stack that up against the damage it could cause to your health (and your waistline) and you'll see that cheesecake will actually get you *further* from your real goal. Fulfilling your dreams requires a healthy heart! It requires taking care of yourself first so you are the best you can be. Once your health is in place and you start having glowing heart health, it becomes so much easier to live from that place. An essential beginning is your diet, and this is something you *can* do something about, but if you are like most people, you probably aren't proactively choosing the foods that are best for your heart (and your butt).

You might have some vague ideas about not eating too much fatty food or junk food or sugar, or you may know a few buzz words like "high-fructose corn syrup" or "trans fat," but many of us do not know exactly what we are really supposed to eat.

One early morning, during the breakfast hour, I was walking to work. You can ask my son about my bad habit of talking to strangers on the street (he thinks I must be personally acquainted with everyone in New York City), but this morning I was in a hurry and I wasn't planning on engaging with anyone at all.

Then I saw a woman wheeling her baby in a stroller and feeding him potato chips, one after the other. He crunched away happily, his little lips and cheeks and chubby fingers smeared with grease. I remember thinking to myself, "Shut up, Suzanne. It's not your business. Don't say a thing."

And then, of course, I did.

I stopped and looked at her. She stopped too, looking uncertain, possibly wondering if she was supposed to know me.

"Why are you feeding your son potato chips for breakfast?" I asked her. "I'm just curious . . . I'm a . . . a . . . cardiologist," I stammered, by way of some sort of justification for butting into this woman's private business.

She looked at me and blinked, a potato chip stalled midway between bag and baby. She probably wanted to tell me that it was none of my business, and of course it wasn't, but then again, the "cardiologist" part had thrown her off guard. She looked at me, and down at the baby, whose chubby hand was reaching for the out-of-reach goody, and then she said, plaintively, with total sincerity, "But these are potatoes! What's so terrible about potatoes?"

I'll spare you the friendly lecture I gave her after that, except to say that she didn't give her baby any more potato chips—at least not until my big mouth and I had turned the next corner and were out of sight.

I tell this story to make a point: I really don't think this perfectly innocent woman knew that what she was doing could possibly have any ill health consequences for her baby. She was thinking: "Potatoes are good for you." She was *not* thinking about how they were fried in cheap oil and doused with salt. That's the problem with thinking: It is selective. It justifies our bad habits. It drowns out our instincts. It picks out the convenient facts and ignores all the others. Meanwhile, her baby was getting indoctrinated at a very young age to love junk food.

I see more extreme examples too.

Jaime, a young professional 23-year-old woman, came into my office recently with supraventricular tachycardia. She was panicking and she asked me, "What's wrong with my heart? Am I going to die?"

"You're not going to die," I assured her. I explained the reasons behind it, and asked her about her life. Was she drinking two pots of coffee a day? Out partying all night?

With a little questioning, I found out that this pretty, well-dressed, just slightly overweight young woman was taking an herbal dietary supplement that was causing her heart to race and its rhythm to become irregular. Also, she was hardly eating anything at all—less than 1,000 calories per day. The herb was an intense appetite suppressant. I've seen this kind of thing before. Some of those herbal supplements can actually cause heart damage after extended use.

She responded with amazement: "But I'm fat! This herb kills my appetite. I'm losing weight. It's working! How can losing weight not be healthier for my heart than being fat?"

She was right that being overweight can be hard on the heart, but what she couldn't seem to see was that the route she was taking to get to a good place was actually leading to a very bad place. This was an intelligent, successful young woman, but all she wanted was for me, her cardiologist, to make the irregular heartbeat go away so she could keep on doing what she wanted to do: take a dangerous diet supplement and keep losing weight. She asked me if I couldn't just give her another pill to fix the side effects from the pill she was already taking. I told her we would find a better way to help her lose weight, but that is not what she wanted.

That's another problem with living from the head. The head is stubborn. It gets an idea and it doesn't want to let go. It doesn't listen to the environmental cues of the body. It doesn't feel. It just rationalizes what it wants to do in the moment.

I could tell you hundreds of stories about how people simply don't realize that what they are doing is harming them, and how stubborn they are about changing their bad habits, and how some don't even believe that their habits are truly bad. It's really not surprising—we live in the information age and we all have access to billions of words that tell us contradictory things about everything that interests us. Whatever you want to do, you can find a statistic or a study or a celebrity to justify it and avoid discomfort.

But discomfort, change, *radical change* are what will be forced upon you if you keep ignoring your heart!

We've become so incredibly removed from what simple healthy living really is that we have no idea how to practice it anymore, and as a result, I see a vast epidemic of cardiac suffering. We've misplaced our instincts about what our bodies need, but we still have them. They are simply buried where we forget to look.

It's my job to help you find your instinct again. You have good instincts. You have intuitions. You can listen to your body's cues, and you should listen to them more than you would listen to some diet plan written by some person who doesn't even know you—myself included!

I *do* happen to know what actual behaviors improve heart health, and I'm going to show them to you in this and upcoming chapters, but I want you to feel them too, not just do what I say because I told you to do it. This is not a prescription. This is simply information. Take the parts that make sense to you, that you feel in your heart are right for you, and then live them.

Step 1: Take Responsibility and Be Accountable

Let's begin right where you are. In order to have an action plan that really works for you, you have to know what you are doing and where your weak spots are. Otherwise you won't know what changes to make. There are several ways to do this. One is a simple personal accounting, which we learned how to do via your own Heart Book.

Now, I am going to ask you to engage your thoughts a bit here. Smart living takes both thinking and feeling, but that doesn't mean I'm putting your brain in charge. Your brain is your heart's personal assistant for now, so keep it in check.

Think about your life and your habits for a few minutes. You probably know exactly which habits are healthful and which are not so much. Start your Heart Book, if you haven't already, so you can begin to be truly accountable for every piece of food you put in your mouth.

Studies show that most people don't actually know how much they eat, and when asked to estimate, almost everyone underestimates portion sizes and leaves off those little bites and bits they grab here and there on the run.

Make no mistake, those bites and bits count! Those portions are what they are! It's time to stop fooling yourself with mental tricks and be open-hearted and honest. You are not doing yourself any favors telling yourself or me that you exercise three to five times a week and hardly eat anything and you don't understand why you are thirty pounds overweight. It's just not possible. If you are thirty pounds overweight, you do *not* exercise three to five times a week, and it is simply *not true* that you hardly eat anything (unless you have some underlying medical condition that needs to be diagnosed, like having a sluggish thyroid).

I can't tell you how often my overweight patients claim that they live "very healthy lifestyles." When I dig for details or demand an accurate food diary from the Heart Book, I see the truth. Patients who think they are eating about 1,500 calories per day are often eating closer to 3,000! Yet they truly believed they were eating 1,500 calories, or even fewer.

It's time for a reality check. Your head may be able to keep you fooled, but your heart knows the truth, and that's where you need to listen.

NO MORE FOOD FANTASIES

I am giving you an assignment. This week, or whenever you are ready to begin taking your health seriously, I want you to begin your Heart Book, or if you have already started it, I want you to be meticulous about writing down every single thing you eat. Every bite.

I mean it. If you finish your child's last two forkfuls of macaroni and cheese, it counts. Write it down. If you find cereal between the couch cushions and you pop it in your mouth (did you really just do that?), it counts. Write it down. You don't have to count up the calories or fat grams or anything like that. No math required. Just write down the content of every single solitary item that goes into your mouth and is swallowed. This, you must do.

Do this on a normal week, or even on a bad week (like a busy or PMS-y week). Don't do this on one of those superhero weeks when you first start a diet or are inspired and doing everything right. How long are you really going to keep that up? If that's not your long-term reality, don't keep your journal during that time. It won't be useful. Save your journaling week for when you fall off the wagon. (Are you already off the wagon and you haven't admitted it to yourself yet? Start writing!)

Be honest with yourself when you are at your worst. If you can fix "at your worst," then when you are at your best, it's easy. Be your regular faulty self with all your food weaknesses, and write it down, write it down, write it down, knowing that you are piecing together your dietary habits in a way that can help you understand them, whether they are good or bad. Facing reality can be painful at first, but it is a temporary and superficial pain. This is good practice for your heart. It doesn't like hiding things. It likes to get the truth out into the open. It's actually a huge relief to fully admit everything you eat. You get to stop living a lie.

But that's not all. We're going to involve your heart even more intimately by doing one more thing, and this is where context comes into play. Whenever you eat, I want you to notice how you feel before, during, and after. Forget the chattering thoughts. Next to your meals, jot down your "feels." You don't have to go on and on about it, just a word or two, like "anxious," "calm," "content," "angry," "tired," "excited," or "a little depressed." This, too, is an excellent process for the upgraded life you are about to embrace.

At the end of the week, I want you to weigh yourself. This is another way to be accountable. Weighing yourself acknowledges the reality of your body as it is right now. It's not good or bad, right or wrong, it's simply reality, and you need to get to know it. Use that number as a tool, not a bludgeon for your self-esteem. Plug it into the BMI chart on page 212 to see where you are: underweight, normal weight, overweight, or obese. No excuses. No "I'm big-boned" or "My family just runs heavy." Accept it for what it is.

Now, you may be wondering about the BMI chart, which has come under fire recently. I've even seen articles in magazines with titles like "BMI? Who Cares!" Well, all I have to say to that is: Your cardiologist cares! I care. The anti-BMI, fat-and-fit movement is a by-product of a culture that keeps getting heavier and wants to justify overweight as the new normal. For example, a size 4 in the United States is a size 8 in Europe. Our sizes keep getting bigger, and we keep putting smaller numbers on them so we can feel better about our expanding shapes.

Belly fat, for example, has been implicated as a serious marker of metabolic risk. A waist circumference of 35 inches or more in a woman (40 inches or more in a man) has been linked to prediabetes and metabolic syndrome. You might be fit, and that's great. It's certainly much, much better than not being fit. However, if you are overweight according to the BMI chart, and you aren't a body builder with an unusual amount of lean muscle, or you don't have gigantic breast implants or some other reason why your weight isn't an accurate representation of your body fat percentage, then the BMI chart is a good indication of where you stand. And ladies, it's quite a range! For example, if you are 5 feet 5 inches tall, you could weigh anywhere from 114 pounds to 150 pounds and still be normal, according to the BMI chart. I think that's pretty lenient. But if you weigh over 150 pounds at 5 feet 5, then face the fact that you will be in better physical condition if you lose some weight.

The point is not to point fingers. The point is not to criticize. The point is certainly not to cause you more stress. I want you to feel compassion for yourself and your body, and start taking steps to feel better now, without getting angry at yourself or feeling frustrated. If you are overweight right now, that is the reality, but it's something you can change. Think of it like a project that you know is going to make you feel great. I want you to be in the best possible shape to avoid heart disease and all the bad things that come along with it.

So let's look at the chart on page 212 and see where you are today.

YOU IN THE MIRROR

Finally, I'd like you to get real with yourself. It's time to take a good, hard look at your body and exactly where you are right now, aside from the journals, the numbers, or anything I say. This is just between you and you.

What physical evidence do you have that your current lifestyle habits are working or not working? Many of us tend to look at our best body parts, or look at ourselves in mirrors in little bits and pieces, avoiding looking at the parts that are in trouble or at the big picture.

Let's peel away another layer of self-delusion. At the end of your week of food recording in your Heart Book, after you weigh yourself, I want you to take a deep breath, find a full-length mirror, lock the door, take off your clothes, and take a good, hard head-to-toe look.

Body Mass Index Table

Body Weight (pounds)

BMI	Normal						Overweight					Obese										Extreme Obesity														
	19	20	21	22	23	24	25	26	27	28	29	30	31	32	33	34	35	36	37	38	39	40	41	42	43	44	45	46	47	48	49	50	51	52	53	54
Height (inches)																																				
58	91	96	100	105	110	115	119	124	129	134	138	143	148	153	158	162	167	172	177	181	186	191	196	201	205	210	215	220	224	229	234	239	244	248	253	258
59	94	99	104	109	114	119	124	128	133	138	143	148	153	158	163	168	173	178	183	188	193	198	203	208	212	217	222	227	232	237	242	247	252	257	262	267
60	97	102	107	112	118	123	128	133	138	143	148	153	158	163	168	174	179	184	189	194	199	204	209	215	220	225	230	235	240	245	250	255	261	266	271	276
61	100	106	111	116	122	127	132	137	143	148	153	158	164	169	174	180	185	190	195	201	206	211	217	222	227	232	238	243	248	254	259	264	269	275	280	285
62	104	109	115	120	126	131	136	142	147	153	158	164	169	175	180	186	191	196	202	207	213	218	224	229	235	240	246	251	256	262	267	273	278	284	289	295
63	107	113	118	124	130	135	141	146	152	158	163	169	175	180	186	191	197	203	208	214	220	225	231	237	242	248	254	259	265	270	278	282	287	293	299	304
64	110	116	122	128	134	140	145	151	157	163	169	174	180	186	192	197	204	209	215	221	227	232	238	244	250	256	262	267	273	279	285	291	296	302	308	314
65	114	120	126	132	138	144	150	156	162	168	174	180	186	192	198	204	210	216	222	228	234	240	246	252	258	264	270	276	282	288	294	300	306	312	318	324
66	118	124	130	136	142	148	155	161	167	173	179	186	192	198	204	210	216	223	229	235	241	247	253	260	266	272	278	284	291	297	303	309	315	322	328	334
67	121	127	134	140	146	153	159	166	172	178	185	191	198	204	211	217	223	230	236	242	249	255	261	268	274	280	287	293	299	306	312	319	325	331	338	344
68	125	131	138	144	151	158	164	171	177	184	190	197	203	210	216	223	230	236	243	249	256	262	269	276	282	289	295	302	308	315	322	328	335	341	348	354
69	128	135	142	149	155	162	169	176	182	189	196	203	209	216	223	230	236	243	250	257	263	270	277	284	291	297	304	311	318	324	331	338	345	351	358	365
70	132	139	146	153	160	167	174	181	188	195	202	209	216	222	229	236	243	250	257	264	271	278	285	292	299	306	313	320	327	334	341	348	355	362	369	376
71	136	143	150	157	165	172	179	186	193	200	208	215	222	229	236	243	250	257	265	272	279	286	293	301	308	315	322	329	338	343	351	358	365	372	379	386
72	140	147	154	162	169	177	184	191	199	206	213	221	228	235	242	250	258	265	272	279	287	294	302	309	316	324	331	338	346	353	361	368	375	383	390	397
73	144	151	159	166	174	182	189	197	204	212	219	227	235	242	250	257	265	272	280	288	295	302	310	318	325	333	340	348	355	363	371	378	386	393	401	408
74	148	155	163	171	179	186	194	202	210	218	225	233	241	249	256	264	272	280	287	295	303	311	319	326	334	342	350	358	365	373	381	389	396	404	412	420
75	152	160	168	176	184	192	200	208	216	224	232	240	248	256	264	272	279	287	295	303	311	319	327	335	343	351	359	367	375	383	391	399	407	415	423	431
76	156	164	172	180	189	197	205	213	221	230	238	246	254	263	271	279	287	295	304	312	320	328	336	344	353	361	369	377	385	394	402	410	418	426	435	443

Source: Adapted from Clinical Guidelines on the Identification, Evaluation, and Treatment of Overweight and Obesity in Adults: The Evidence Report. Taken from the National Heart Lung and

Look at everything. The strong muscles. The pockets of fat. The beautiful facial structure. The lumpy cellulite. The nice hair. The muffin top. Do you have back fat? Gorgeous eyes? Knee dimples? Strong biceps? Mentally note your greatest features, and also mentally note where you've let yourself go. Try to be objective. It won't be easy, but this is tough love, because when your body is heavy with excess adipose tissue (translation: FAT!), you need to acknowledge that.

I don't want this to be a depressing exercise, although many people will feel a bit overwhelmed or defeated doing this. However, I want you to have a serious reality check. Body type is one thing. We all have different shapes, and I want you to love your natural shape. But can you see your natural shape anymore? Where did it go? If your body has been a war zone after years of overeating and neglect, it has paid a price for the way you treat it, and I want you to look that reality square in the face. Your naturally muscular calves are *fine*. Your freckles are *gorgeous*. Your broad shoulders are *regal*. But that thigh or hip or stomach fat? That is putting your health and happiness at risk, and that is something you can do something about.

I wish you could also see your heart during this exercise. I wish you could see your arteries, and whether they are stiff and fatty or clean and flexible. There is something extraordinarily life-changing about looking at a heart in the operating room. Before a bypass, in those patients who have a buildup of plaque in the arteries, there is fat surrounding the heart. This yellow, thick coating on your heart, impeding its ability to work at peak efficiency, is something to think about before you pop that French fry into your mouth. What you see on the outside is only a reflection of the inside.

So just get naked and stand in front of the mirror. Bright lights and all.

And you thin women, don't think you are exempt. Even women who are thin on the outside may have fatty tissue and stiff arteries, depending on how they eat and move and live, so just because the mirror shows you a thin person doesn't mean you are totally off the hook. Not just yet.

Now, enough thinking! Let's involve your heart. Let it feel love for your body, maybe some grief for your suffering, and certainly hope for your future. I want you to feel the glow of your own personality, your kindness, your beautiful uniqueness. I want you to feel deep, genuine compassion for yourself.

Then I want you to make your mirror image a promise:

I promise I will do what's best for you, from now on!

Promise your heart, promise your body, promise your mind, promise yourself. And then . . . let's take action!

Heart Sense

High blood pressure is one of the best known and most serious heart disease risks, and one of the biggest influences on blood pressure is dietary sodium. Most people should get about 2,100 milligrams of sodium per day, and that's not very much, especially if you eat processed foods. If you have high blood pressure, diabetes, or kidney disease, you should limit your intake to about 1,500 milligrams.

The problem isn't usually the salt shaker. It's the foods in the packages. There are ten kinds of foods that make up 44 percent of the sodium content we eat each day, and the saltiest versions are most likely to be packaged store-bought food or restaurant foods. Sodium is most concentrated in bread, cold cuts and cured meats, pizza, poultry (chicken and turkey, which often have salt added), soups, sandwiches, cheese, pasta mixed dishes, meat mixed dishes, and packaged snacks. If you eliminated these foods, just by staying away from packaged foods and eating less restaurant food (or asking for your food to be prepared without salt), your high blood pressure would likely go down.

Or just reduce your sodium intake by about one-fourth. If everyone did that, that alone could prevent 28,000 deaths and 7 billion dollars in health-care costs every year.

Step 2: Analyze This

The next step is to analyze what you've written in your Heart Book over the past week. Read back over it all. Does it sound like what you thought you were eating? Do you find any surprises? Are you thinking to yourself, "Did I really eat all that?" This is a time to engage your brain again. Look for patterns. Look for favorite foods. Look for the things you just can't stop eating. Don't do this with guilt, but with objectivity, as if you were looking at someone else's food journal. Where are your obvious weaknesses? If you could edit this journal, what would you change, just based on your instincts?

You can also show your journal to a healthy friend (one of your more straightforward friends) for a second opinion. What do your food choices look like to her? Sometimes it's easier for someone else to see where we are falling down.

You will probably notice that you tend to gravitate toward certain foods. Almost everyone does. Maybe you are a crunchy-salty person, or a creamy-sweet person, or a chocolate person, or a cheese-and-crackers or nachos person. Almost everyone has a food weakness. You know who you are.

I've found that for most people, generally the weakness is either primarily about carbohydrates or fat. It doesn't mean you won't also enjoy other foods. A chocolate addict may also have her potato chip moments. Some people have to have French fries, but they are happy to chase them down with a milk shake. Looking over your food diary, figure out where your real weaknesses lie. Ask yourself if it's that sweet taste that moves you, or whether it's the fat or salt that you crave. Do you love everything fried (like Buffalo wings and fried fish), or just fried starch (like French fries and doughnuts)? Do you have to have sugar, even if it's in a nonfat form like Skittles or jellybeans? Are you more about the bread or the butter?

Earlier in this book, I recommended that you get an ApoE test (I explained what this is in Chapters 2 and 8). This genetic test can determine whether you have more trouble metabolizing carbohydrates or more trouble metabolizing fat (about 65 percent of people are able to metabolize both without a problem). In my experience with hundreds of patients, I have noticed that those who have the genotype that has trouble metabolizing carbs are the very ones who crave and binge on carbs like cookies, jellybeans, bread, and soda. Those who have the genotype that can't metabolize fat efficiently are the very ones who can't stop eating the Buffalo wings, cheeseburgers, nachos, and rich ice cream. I can also often tell by other tests. If your LDL cholesterol is high, then often fat in the diet is the culprit. If your triglycerides are elevated, then carbohydrates may be your issue.

Know your dietary Achilles' heel. But here's the good news: You can make your dietary preferences work for you by only slightly tweaking your choices.

Your Heart

I had a patient come in the other day who had an elevated LDL cholesterol, despite dieting. She'd been eating a low-carb diet, and she didn't understand why it wasn't working. I did an ApoE test on her, and we found she had one ApoE3 gene and one ApoE4 gene.

I told her, "You can't eat meat. You can't digest fat."

"You just changed my entire life," she said.

Sometimes people decide to go low-carb, or on the other end of the spectrum, vegetarian, not realizing that a particular diet just isn't right for them because they can't metabolize fat or they can't metabolize sugar and carbohydrates. When you are planning your diet, the ApoE test can make a big difference in what you decide to do for yourself, so especially if you have high triglycerides or high cholesterol, ask your doctor about this test before you completely change your diet.

Step 3: Change One Thing

Change is hard—especially drastic change. So let's not do that. Let's stick with what you can actually handle. Now that you know your weak spots, let's work on your one weakest area. It's so much easier than taking on all your bad habits at once. Improve this one thing, and you will be taking a big leap forward for your health and well-being. Behavioral patterns are hard to break, so the trick is to fit a healthier choice into the same behavior pattern, at least at first. For example, if you sit down with potato chips or corn chips in front of the TV every evening, and you genuinely can't imagine not doing that, that's where you have to start. Could you snack on apple slices with low-fat cheese? Whole-grain pretzels? Pistachios, which require peeling and slow you down? Baked chips? What about a few stalks of crunchy celery with some peanut butter? Instead of denying yourself an evening snack or the (mind-numbing) television experience, start by snacking smarter.

I have some patients who drink so much soda, it truly shocks me. I had one patient tell me, "But it's okay because it's ginger ale!" I just had to sigh and shake my head. If you are a soda drinker and you just can't imagine ever giving that up, ask yourself what it is about soda that you love. Is it the bubbles? The sweet taste? Could you switch to club soda with a splash of real juice and start there? Another common bad habit I see is the patient who has to have something sweet or starchy in the morning, like a muffin, sugary cereal, or bagel. Starchy breakfasts filled with simple sugars might perk you up for an hour or two, but they are also likely to cause a midafternoon crash because they set your blood sugar on a wild ride. When breakfast is a simple sugar, like a doughnut, for example, your blood sugar rises too quickly. To combat this imbalance, your insulin kicks in and your blood sugar drops, and then you feel like you need another fix. If you tend to get that 3:00 p.m. crash—you know, the one that can only be remedied by more sugar or a trip to the nearest coffee shop, where you say yes to the whipped cream on that coffee drink—evaluate what you had for breakfast. This is where your day really begins.

If this sounds like you but you can't imagine giving up your starchy breakfast, think about how you can eat your beloved carbohydrates without sending your blood sugar on a roller-coaster ride. The key is not to avoid all carbs but to choose low glycemic–index foods.

The glycemic index is an index that essentially ranks foods according to simple sugar content and how quickly the food is metabolized. High-glycemic foods make blood sugar rise very quickly, while low-glycemic foods keep the blood sugar lower and steadier. Whenever I say to minimize "carbs," what I really mean is to minimize high-glycemic foods. For example, white bread, white pasta, bagels, white rice, white potatoes, corn, and bananas are high-glycemic foods. You might notice that white and light yellow foods tend to be high-glycemic, and this is true! In most cases, avoid white foods! Whole grains, vegetables, and some high-fiber fruits are low-glycemic foods. Fiber slows down the sugar uptake in the bloodstream so your blood sugar stays steadier and you don't get ravenous a few hours after eating.

What this means for your breakfast is that you should start the day with protein, which also keeps blood sugar steady, and whole grains, like a whole-wheat English muffin with peanut butter, an egg-white omelet with wheat toast, or Greek yogurt with berries and a little bit of whole-grain high-fiber cereal mixed in. You'll get that starchy taste, but the protein and fiber will slow down the release of sugar into your blood. You'll feel calmer and more stable and you won't be jonesing for candy or a caramel macchiato in the afternoon. Changing your one worst thing can have a dramatic impact. It may feel like a slow start, much less dramatic and promising than going on a diet (I hate that four-letter word!), but I've seen it make a big impact. When my patients alter their one worst habit and do nothing else, they often drop twenty pounds, just like that. That's not to say that giving up your worst dietary sin is easy. It's not. You're going to want those chips, that soda, the giant muffin, the afternoon candy bar, just out of habit, but if you choose something else instead, if you forgo your fix, guess what?

You are not going to die.

I tell my patients this frequently. *You are not going to die!* At least not today. You might feel like you want to die if you can't have that muffin, but in reality, you are only mildly upset. Your body is throwing a toddler's temper tantrum because it can't have what it is used to getting. I also tell my patients that they may not like breaking their worst habit, but they can take it out on me. Blame the cardiologist. Shake your fist at me all day long if you like. Give me the finger; I can take it. I've had cab drivers do worse. In a week, when your craving has weakened, and then in six weeks when your craving is totally gone, you'll be thanking me because of how much better you feel.

Heart Sense

For a while, I was getting weekly calls from the media to discuss dark chocolate, red wine, or coffee. I was a little worried that I would get typecast as the Cardiologist of Vice! This is what you should know about how they affect your heart:

Chocolate: The bioflavonoids and polyphenols found in dark chocolate can help lower blood pressure, improve endothelial function, reduce inflammation, decrease the development of blood clots, prevent weight gain, stabilize blood sugar, and prevent cardiovascular disease. Chocolate that contains 70 percent cocoa is the most effective, because it has the greatest amount of polyphenols and bioflavonoids, which lead to the release of nitric oxide and dilatation of the arteries. I eat one to two squares of 70 percent dark chocolate every day, and I recommend that you do too. Consider it a prescription. Doctor's orders!

Alcohol: Red wine is filled with the same polyphenols as chocolate. These flavonoids do the same fabulous things that chocolate does—reduce inflammation, prevent blood clots, dilate the arteries, decrease the bad cholesterol, and increase the good. Red wine (specifically Bordeaux) is highest in these flavonoids, and is best for the heart. Other wines and spirits are also beneficial, but not quite the powerhouse that red wine is. Red wine also contains resveratrol, which is the nonflavonoid antioxidant that prevents the arteries from becoming clogged by preventing clotting, decreasing inflammation, dilating the arteries, and decreasing LDL cholesterol. Resveratrol is on the skin of grapes, and because red wine is fermented with grape skins longer than white wine is, red wine has more resveratrol. The general recommendation is one drink per day for women and two for men. But that is just a four- to five-ounce glass.

I'm not talking a huge goblet full! If you drink too much, you can increase your risk of high blood pressure, high triglycerides, obesity, cancer, and liver damage. It can cause an irregular heartbeat like atrial fibrillation or dilate the heart by weakening the heart muscle. If you like wine, find your happy medium and stay there. Drinking too much is worse than not drinking at all.

Coffee and tea: People who drink two to four cups of coffee a day compared to those who drink less than two and greater than four cups per day have a 20 percent reduction of heart disease. Coffee is controversial, and it can potentially contribute to the development of breast cancer, so moderation is key. Regarding tea, those people who drank more than six cups of tea a day had a 36 percent decreased risk of heart disease compared to those who drank less than one cup per day, and those who drank three to six cups had a 45 percent reduced risk of heart disease, so it seems like three to six cups may be where the tea sweet spot is. Just watch out for the effects of caffeine. It can increase your heart rate, causing extra beats, and can also increase your blood pressure.

I had a patient whom I'll call Tony. Tony was a big meat eater. Steak, pork, chicken wings, meatloaf, burgers—this was his dietary nirvana, and his dietary weakness. He considered himself a low-carb dieter, and he was only slightly overweight, but his cholesterol was off the charts, and I strongly suspected he was one of those people who could not metabolize fat very well.

I told him he had to stop. Stop doing it, I said. Stop with the meat. He looked at me in horror, but I reassured him: In a few weeks, you won't even want it anymore. Six weeks later, he came back to my office, and he'd dropped ten pounds, he had more energy, and the thought of a greasy hunk of meat turned his stomach.

If you hang in there, doctor's orders, it will happen for you too. You're not as hopeless as you think. It's just *one* bad habit.

Your Dietary Achilles' Heel

IF YOU:	THEN TRY:
Crunch away in front of the TV	Mini rice cakes
	Air-popped popcorn
	Whole-grain pretzels (but watch the salt and stick to one portion)
	Celery with peanut butter
	Portion-controlled nuts
	Nuts or seeds with shells, like pistachios and sunflower seeds
Drink soda	Club soda with splash of fresh juice
	Fruit chunks in mineral water
Eat sweet or starchy breakfasts	Egg-white omelet and whole-grain toast
	Whole-grain English muffin with nut butter
	Oatmeal with flax seeds and blueberries
	Greek yogurt with berries and whole-grain high-fiber cereal
	Low-fat cottage cheese with berries and sliced almonds

Crave candy midafternoon	Eating protein at every meal
	Apple with almond butter
	Green drink with apple juice added
	Plain Greek yogurt with blueberries and 1 teaspoon mini chocolate chips
	A handful of nuts
	Berries, apples, pears
	High-fiber protein bar

Step 4: Make a Rule and Live It

Finally, I want you to start eating better in general. I don't want you to go on a diet. I just want you to start making better choices, choices that will directly affect how you feel and how you live and how you look too.

The best way I've found to do this is to make a rule and stick with it. You've kicked your worst bad habit. Now figure out something you can live with that is more general and applies to your whole day.

To give you some ideas, I'll list some of my favorite effective dietary principles here. Choose a rule, choose two or three. Then live them.

The beauty of choosing a rule versus following a diet is that a rule can go with you anywhere. You can go out to eat. You can visit with friends. You can go to happy hour. You can cook a cool recipe you saw in a magazine. As long as you follow your rule *most* of the time, you'll be moving in the right direction.

Dr. Steinbaum's Dietary Rules for Life

A few good rules are worth a hundred diet books. Here are the rules I believe are most beneficial for heart and overall physical and mental health. Start with the ones that seem the most doable, and work up from there. If you are practicing all of these tactics, eventually you'll be on the fast track to fabulous. For now, just start with one or two and work your way up:

- No high-glycemic foods ever, and as few carbohydrate-rich foods (grains, fruit, anything with sugar) as possible after 3:00 p.m. If you eat a vegetarian diet, load up on vegetables and beans, and save your grains for morning. This one rule alone will likely cause you to drop most of your excess weight. I swear by it. It really works. You need the quick energy from carbohydrates during the day when you are busy, but at night when you are winding down, they aren't necessary, so this rule helps you eat in tune with your body's needs. Stick to protein and vegetables (like grilled salmon, tofu, or chicken with sautéed green beans or broccoli and salad) and you'll be amazed at how quickly you lose weight and feel better.

- Breakfast must include a complex carbohydrate and a protein. Examples: an egg-white omelet with all the vegetables you want and multigrain toast, or multigrain toast with a slice of low-fat cheese and a slice of tomato, or Greek yogurt with fruit and granola. Eat as many vegetables as you can possibly get into your system at any opportunity. I call this being "as vegetarian as possible."

- Never, ever drink soda, regular or diet.

- Never eat more than one sugar-containing item per day, maximum. One or two squares of dark chocolate is the perfect dessert, but if you must, one small scoop of ice cream, one small cookie, or just a bite or two of a larger pastry. Take your pick.

- Incorporate omega-3s into your diet. Either eat fish two to three times a week; incorporate canola oil, olive oil, or flaxseed oil into your diet; or take a daily supplement.

There now—is that so hard? These are changes anyone can practice most of the time, no four-letter D-word required.

This Chapter by Heart

♥ Consider what you really want. What is masquerading as a desire for food?

♥ In your Heart Book, keep a totally honest accounting of what you eat for at least one week. Examine it for patterns.

♥ At the end of the week, weigh yourself, and take a good, hard look at yourself in the mirror, with compassion.

♥ Based on your Heart Book, decide what your one worst dietary habit is, and work on changing it by substituting something healthier.

♥ Choose one or two new rules for yourself, and stick to them, no matter what.

CHAPTER TEN

Exercise: The Ultimate Prescription

Having spent a lifetime exercising, I have an enormous appreciation for how exercise can make you feel. Throughout my busy
life, I have always tried on some level to keep active and to keep moving. At one point, I took dance classes five days a week, which then
led to going to the gym four days a week, which morphed into an
exercise class three days a week, which then led to an elliptical trainer
and disco dancing in my apartment with my son. Regardless of my life
situation and circumstances, I know firsthand what it feels like to
exercise and what it feels like not to exercise. I also know firsthand
that the key to vitality, longevity, and the fountain of youth is exercise. I get to see that every day with my patients. And, quite frankly,
I admire the women whose exercise routines make them appear ten to
twenty years younger than they are. Their hearts, minds, and overall
wellness all benefit immeasurably from regular exercise.

Exercise is such a significant part of my existence that when I had
shoulder surgery recently, I realized how crucial it was for me to get
my body moving to get me back to myself. I knew that no matter how
busy I was, I had to make time for physical therapy (see my physical

therapist Luke's heart on page 176), and then after work at night, I would continue to do the exercises and stretches. My son, Spencer, would do them with me every day. One night as I was putting him to bed, after a long day of work and a night of trying to skip the program, he said, "Mommy, let's stretch before we go to bed." Even he knew that we'd both feel better with a bit of exercise and stretching each day. Then he jumped down onto the floor and started stretching his shoulder and then trying to touch his toes, making a little grunting noise. (Of course, my first thought was: "Do I do that?") He also has taken to wearing a pedometer to school just to see which one of us takes more steps each day. That was his idea. I swear.

I've managed to teach my son how important exercise is to life, and now I want to teach you. I know the transformative power of exercise. I have seen it heal hearts, restore vitality, effect weight loss, improve mood, and generally make people dramatically healthier.

Healthy people get exercise. Period. I'm not going to argue about this. It's simply true. In a meta-analysis of thirty-three trials involving exercise and death rates among 187,000 healthy men and women, higher levels of cardiorespiratory fitness were associated with a lower risk of death from all causes during any given study period. When my patients do well on a stress test, I know they are less likely to get sick or be sick, and when they do poorly, I expect the opposite. It's a direct correlation.

However, the simple fact is that 60 percent of American men and women over thirty-five are physically inactive. This is a great way to escort heart disease into your life, and I wish I could impress upon every single person in this country how important it is to exercise to save your heart. Exercise helps you to improve your Heart Throbs almost across the board. It helps to lower your blood pressure, reduce your cholesterol, lower your body weight, and improve your mood. Exercise alone, independent of all other Heart Throbs, decreases your risk of heart disease, and in many studies, those who exercised, which included simply regular walking, were much less likely to die from any cause. Exercise can help to prevent cognitive decline and Alzheimer's disease, cancer, metabolic syndrome, and diabetes, and it makes you feel great because of the serotonin (the feel-good hormone) release that happens during exercise.

When I was going through a difficult time in my life a few years ago and went for a long time without exercise, I remember the horrible feeling of not being able to breathe very well. I was becoming deconditioned, and as a former dancer, I'd never felt like that before. There is something extremely dramatic and frightening about that feeling. If you've never been fit, you don't necessarily realize what you are missing, but if you have been fit, your body knows exactly how much it wants to get back to that place. When I started exercising again, my fitness level went back up quickly because my body remembered what it was like to be in shape. Even if you stop exercising for a long period, you can start again and it will come back to you.

The longer you can sustain an exercise routine, the more forgiving your body will be in the event that you can't exercise for a while, such as when you go on vacation, have a particularly stressful time at work, need surgery, go through childbirth, or just plain get too busy. When you return to exercise (like returning to an old friend), your muscles and your heart will start smiling, and it will take a much shorter time to get back into it. You just have to restart.

We are all human. Things happen. Just don't give up. Every time you restart, it gets easier, and it's *never* too late. Exercise will always welcome you back. I can't think of one good reason not to do it.

What Is Exercise?

Exercise is movement that creates an energy demand in your body. The kind of exercise that is best for your heart is "cardio," or the type that increases your heart rate for a sustained period of time. In Chapter 8, I told you a little bit about the stress test, but just to quickly review, this is the common way doctors evaluate fitness. You begin on a treadmill, walking at a low level of METs. Remember METs? That's the measurement of how much oxygen is required or energy needed to perform an exercise. The higher the METs, the greater the effort.

As the treadmill goes faster and the incline gets steeper, the METs increase. Based on your age, you should be able to reach a certain METs number before reaching your target heart rate. If you fall below it, you are not fit. If you reach it, you are "normal." If you take even longer to get to your target heart rate, that means your heart doesn't have to work very hard at all, even when you are exercising, and that means you are in great shape.

This is the whole point of cardiovascular exercise: to get your heart into good shape so it doesn't have to pump very hard when you exert yourself. The stronger your heart, the easier physical activity will be, and the more fit you are. When patients come into my office and do a stress test, I often tell them their results by explaining to them where they are on the scale of being physically fit, and what their goal should be. Then we figure out exactly how they are going to get there. You can do this for yourself. My patients often wonder if they are in shape, and there are ways you can determine this on your own without ever taking a stress test. Once you know your fitness level, you can set a goal and work toward it. You can write your own exercise prescription.

STEP 1: DETERMINE YOUR TARGET HEART RATE

Your target heart rate is the heart rate at which you should be exercising. A lot of people who exercise don't do it vigorously enough, and some people overdo it. When you know your target heart rate, you can exercise for maximum fitness. Figure out your target heart rate with this simple calculation:

(220 − your age) x .85 = _____

This is the target heart rate for someone who is not sick and is in fairly good shape. If you are sick or you know you haven't exercised in a very long time, use this calculation instead, but consider the number above to be your ultimate goal:

(220 − your age) x .50 = _____

Now you have your *target heart rate*.

So what do you do with this information?

STEP 2: GET A HEART MONITOR, OR LEARN HOW TO ASSESS YOUR PERCEIVED EXERTION

A heart monitor is one of the most valuable tools you can have, and if you make the investment, use it every time you exercise. Now that you know your target heart rate, your goal when exercising is to keep your heart at your target heart rate for 30 sustained minutes. You might not be able to do this at first. You might have to work up to 30 minutes, and that's okay. As long as you are working toward your goal, you are still exercising. Your sustained 30 minutes does not count warming up and cooling down, when your heart rate should be below your target heart rate.

A heart monitor is an excellent way to be sure you are working out hard enough to benefit your heart. If your heart rate goes below the zone indicated on the monitor, then you know you need to pick up the pace! (If it goes above the zone, don't worry. You aren't going to spontaneously combust. It just means you are working extra hard, and unless you already know you have a heart issue that precludes exercise, this is just fine for your heart.)

If you can't or don't want to buy a heart monitor, there is an alternate way to figure out how vigorously you should be exercising. It's called rate of perceived exertion, or RPE. One way to measure this is through the Borg Scale of Physical Activity.

Basically, the Borg Scale tells us what our perceived exertion is during any given activity. The scale goes from 6 to 20 (don't ask me why), and we used it when I was seeing patients in cardiac rehab, because some of our patients were on medication that kept their heart rates low and therefore the target heart rate formula didn't apply. This was a more accurate way to perceive their exertion during exercise.

The Borg Scale helps you to determine for yourself how hard you are working. No effort, such as sitting doing nothing, would be rated a 6. If you would describe your effort as light, your rating would be 11 to 12. Moderate effort would be 13 to 14, as you might feel with brisk walking. You can still talk, but you might not be able to sing. Hard effort would be a 15 to 16 and would get your heart pounding. You might have trouble finishing your sentences at this level. Very hard would be at your greatest sustainable effort, rated 17 to 18. A 19 or 20 would be a level of effort that you could do in short spurts, like a sprint, but that you could not sustain for more than a few minutes.

The level on the Borg Scale that would correspond to your target heart rate (using the .85 calculation from Step 1) would be at about 13 to 15. That's where you want to exercise for 30 sustained minutes.

STEP 3: CALCULATE YOUR METS

Unlike the Borg Scale, METs are based not on perceived exertion but on how much oxygen your body actually uses during various levels of activity. This is how cardiologists assess your fitness. Honestly, it's also a somewhat arbitrary scale, but this is the measure we use to determine physical fitness, or as I call it, cardiac vitality.

During a stress test, we do not expect a fit person to reach her target heart rate until she has reached the MET level expected for her age. Calculate your MET level with this formula:

14.7 − (.13 x your age) = _____

Now, let's say you are 40 years old. Your target heart rate used for a stress test is:

(220 − 40) x .87 = 156.6

That means you want to get your heart rate up to about 156 to 157 and keep it there for 30 minutes about 5 days per week.

Your MET level is 14.7 − (.13 x 40) = 9.5

Now, what does that mean? That means that when you exercise, your heart should not reach 156 beats per minute until you are exercising at a MET level of 9.5.

You can find a lot of lists that estimate MET level for various activities, but a more accurate way to determine what MET level corresponds to how hard you are working is to use an exercise machine, like a treadmill, that has a MET readout. If you are 40 years old and you go to the gym and start jogging on the treadmill wearing your heart monitor and your heart rate reaches 156 when you are only running at 7 METs, then that means you are out of shape.

This is exactly what we do on a stress test. The treadmills we use calculate METs, and we see what MET level gets you to your target heart rate. If you are 40, we hope you won't get there until you hit 9.5 METs. If you are out of shape, that probably won't happen. If you are in great shape, you might not reach your target heart rate until you hit 10 or 12 METs.

I used to give stress tests to the New York Knicks, and not only did we have to alter the test somewhat because they were in such great shape that it was hard to get them to their target heart rates (and they had such long legs that running on our treadmills was easy for them), but we actually had to remove some of the ceiling tiles so they wouldn't bump their heads on our ceiling!

But you probably are not in quite as good shape as the New York Knicks.

Or maybe you are? Would you like to see? Would you like to give yourself a stress test?

You can actually do this with a treadmill on your own if you use something we call the Bruce Protocol. This is how we adjust the treadmill in a real stress test. This will show you exactly how you would score, so you can assess whether or not a cardiologist would deem you fit.

Here's how you do it. Just promise me you won't try this at home if you have any symptoms of heart disease or any worrisome Heart Throbs. In that case, you have to go to your doctor first and get approval to start exercising. Before you read ahead, just promise me that.

STEP 4: GIVE YOURSELF A STRESS TEST

Strap on your heart monitor, then head to that treadmill. You don't even need one that records METs. All you need is the Bruce Protocol.

The Bruce Protocol is what we use to determine METs. Start the treadmill at the indicated speed and grade or incline. Each stage lasts for 3 minutes. As you walk and run, keep track of your heart rate. When you reach your target heart rate, stop. The stage at which you stopped indicates the METs you achieved. Remember, you are hoping to reach your age-expected METs (which you calculated in the previous step) before you reach your target heart rate (which you also calculated before). Also, I want you to understand that this is a starting point for fitness. The longer it takes you to reach your target heart rate while working at your age-expected METs level, the fitter you are. Are you ready? Turn on the treadmill:

STAGE 1:   1.7 mph, 10% grade, 4–5 METs: 3 minutes

STAGE 2:   2.5 mph, 12% grade, 7–8 METs: 3 minutes

STAGE 3: 3.4 mph, 14% grade, 9–10 METs: 3 minutes

STAGE 4: 4.2 mph, 16% grade, 12–13 METs: 3 minutes

STAGE 5: 5.0 mph, 18% grade, 15–16 METs: 3 minutes

STAGE 6: 5.5 mph, 20% grade, over 16 METs: 3 minutes

You can go higher, but most people I see don't ever get beyond stage 6 (except those guys from the Knicks!).

This is just one of eight different treadmill protocols you can find out there, but this is the most common one used in the United States, so if you do ever have to have a stress test, these probably are the numbers your doctor will use.

So how did you do? Are you fit? Or do you need some work?

STEP 5: GIVE YOURSELF AN EXERCISE PRESCRIPTION

According to American Heart Association guidelines, you should be doing one of the following:

- 150 minutes of moderate-intensity exercise a week, or about 30 minutes 5 days per week. Moderate-intensity exercise means about 8 or 9 METs, or 13 to 15 on the Borg Scale. You could talk to the person next to you with some effort, but you couldn't sing.

or

- 75 minutes of vigorous-intensity aerobic activity. Vigorous-intensity exercise means you can't really finish a sentence very easily. You are huffing and puffing! This would be 10 to 12 METs, or 16 to 18 on the Borg Scale. That's just 15 minutes 5 days per week, or 25 minutes 3 days per week.

In addition to cardiovascular activity, I would also like you to do:

- Strength training, focusing on your major muscle groups. Do 1 to 2 sets of 10 to 15 reps 2 or 3 days every week. If you work your major muscles, like your quadriceps, biceps, abdominals, and gluteus (butt) muscles, you will burn more calories even when you aren't doing anything, and that can help fight both diabetes and obesity. You don't have to go to the gym. Buy some inexpensive resistance bands or a set of hand weights to keep at home. You can even use water jugs as weights.

If you have that heart rate monitor, make sure you stay at your target heart rate, or gradually work up to it, increasing your effort just a little bit each week. This all might sound like a lot right now, but don't let these numbers intimidate you. Remember, you are taking back control of your life, and all you have to do is start. If there is no way you can fit in that 30 minutes at one time, do 10-minute increments 3 times per day (you should always exercise for at least 10 minutes at any given time to receive any benefit). Go up and down the stairs for 10 minutes every morning and evening. During the middle of the day, do it again at your job. It could be the first part of your lunch break. Keep pushing yourself just enough that you see improvement but not so much that you get frustrated and give up. Work up to it, then keep it up. Regularity is more important than intensity. Just do something, even if it doesn't seem like much at first. Believe it or not, once you are in the habit, exercise feels so good that you won't want to miss it. In fact, my goal is to get you to that level where you will do almost anything *not* to miss your daily exercise. I want you to crave that feeling of moving, breathing, sweating, and the scrotonin release (happy hormone!) that accompanies it.

The Many Ways to Exercise

One of the easiest, totally free, enjoyable ways to exercise is walking. Keep the pace brisk, and put a pedometer on every day, with the goal of reaching at least 10,000 steps. If you see you're behind in the middle of the day, then you just might have to walk a little more to catch up, but if you can't make it to the swimming pool, tennis court, or gym that day, at least you know that you have achieved a level of exercise recommended by the American Heart Association.

Some people like the gym. I'm not a fan, but if you are, enjoy any of those cardio machines. Many of them have their own personal magazine stands and even televisions, so you can watch TV while you exercise. That thirty minutes will fly by if you're watching your favorite show. Or get a personal trainer to show you some moves, and go from there.

Heart Sense

Interval training is a kind of exercise where the heart rate is pushed to its maximum level, then decreased, through periods of extreme exertion alternating with periods of less exertion. Interval training can be an excellent way to exercise, as long as the periods of lower intensity or exertion are brief, so the heart rate doesn't come down too much. If the heart rate drops below the 75th percentile, then you're not getting maximum cardiovascular benefit. This defeats the purpose of exercising for heart health.

But walking and the gym aren't your only options. You can exercise outdoors or indoors, at home or on the job. You can walk, jog, run, sprint, jump rope, or do calisthenics. You can lift weights, do yoga or Pilates, or do sit-ups, push-ups, and jumping jacks in front of the (mind-numbing) television every night. If you want to play golf, forget the cart and the caddy. Walk and carry your clubs. If you commute, take the stairs to and from the train. You can also just be active. Living in New York City, many people are in better shape than those in some other parts of the country because it is a walking city. People walk everywhere, and they don't just meander or stroll. They walk quickly and with purpose. They are up and down the stairs that lead in and out of the subway. Many are fit without having a formal exercise program.

When I have patients who live in the city and use their feet as their transportation, many of them do very well on a stress test. But even if you don't live in a walking city, you can still walk. Carry your heels and put on your tennis shoes and walk everywhere you can. I don't care if you're wearing a dress. You don't have to wear workout clothes. You don't have to get drenched in sweat. Just walk! Maybe walking will graduate to jogging, jogging to running, and then maybe you will need some sweatpants, but don't worry about that now if you're not ready for it. Maybe you'll do it on a treadmill or in a park, or maybe you'll just walk the local mall. You can also take the stairs instead of the elevator or escalator. You can park farther away. You can do squats while you wait for the water on the stove to boil or arm circles while your bath is filling up. You can take out the trash and do a few bicep curls with the trash bags. You can do high kicks just for fun. You can join your kids on the playground instead of sitting on the park bench. And you can always put on some music and dance. (Kids *love* it when Mommy dances!)

It all depends on your life, and if you don't fit exercise into the reality of your life, then it's never going to stick. Just keep moving. Just being active and moving around a lot has the same effect on your body as exercise if you do it vigorously enough. You could be knitting and doing leg lifts at the same time and be getting a great workout, as opposed to meandering around the block at a leisurely pace that doesn't raise your heart rate or work your muscles very much.

I don't want you to think that if you are going to exercise, you have to do it one way. I just want you to do it *some* way.

When Spencer was a newborn, I didn't want to leave him to go exercise. But that didn't stop me because I knew how important it was for me. I held him and did plies, or turned on disco and danced all around my apartment with him (we still do this). He was singing "Shake your booty" by the age of two. To me this was about cardiovascular survival, sustaining health, and being a good mom. Sometimes I used him as a weight to do chest presses and bicep curls. All of this counts! You just have to move.

I know that for many people, the notion of exercise is intimidating. When you aren't in the habit, it's a mighty hard habit to form, but if you don't exercise, things aren't going well inside your chest, I can assure you. I can confirm deconditioning with a stress test in my office, but I can often tell without the test when someone is huffing and puffing just to climb onto the exam table.

The simple fact is that your heart is a muscle, and if you don't exercise it, it's going to get deconditioned, just like your biceps or your quadriceps would become deconditioned if you didn't use them enough. When the heart gets deconditioned, it becomes more demanding in its needs, less functional, and less able to do its job. Effort will be harder for your heart. It will have to pump hard just to help you walk across the room or climb a flight of stairs. Your heart shouldn't have to do that. You need all your muscles in good working condition, but none more than your heart if you want to keep moving and thinking and working and, oh, I don't know, *staying alive*? But you don't want to just survive, do you? You want to thrive. You want to be strong, energized, graceful, capable, independent, and vital well into old age. That takes a little bit of work.

The human body is meant to move, and move a lot. Why do you think we have all those muscles and joints? Exercise is the ultimate prescription. No matter what your fitness level, no matter what your health issues, it is almost *always* okay to get a little more exercise than you are getting now. And then a little more. And then a little more.

This is why I encourage you to start where you are. You don't have to go out and run a marathon. If all you can do is walk around the block, then today get up and walk around the block. *Just do something.*

Regularity is more important than time or intensity.

Don't judge yourself against anyone else or anyone's guidelines. Just get up and do something. Movement is life. Stasis is death. Move, ladies and gentlemen! Move it or lose it, and I mean that literally!

Heart Sense

People tend to have an all-or-nothing attitude. They will exercise every day for a few days, but when they miss a day, they think they've blown it and then they skip another week or two. This is a mistake, because when you stop exercising for too long, your progress starts reversing and you become deconditioned again.

But not right away! Here is my rule of thumb, and it's the most important thing to remember in this chapter:

Never go for more than two days without exercise.

If you have a good exercise session but then you miss exercise the next day, don't despair. Just get back on it. You won't lose any ground as long as you don't go for more than two days without it.

As you progress in your exercise journey, I recommend monitoring your progress so you can be sure you are really getting your heart rate where it needs to be to actually get all the benefits.

A good start is to record your exercise in your Heart Book. Write down what you did, and for how long. If you use a heart monitor, write down your numbers. If you are keeping track of your perceived exertion or your METs, write that down too. Write down how you did on your stress test. Write down your exercise prescription and check off every day that you fill that prescription. When you look back over your Heart Book in a few months, it will be so rewarding to see how far you've come—from ten or fifteen minutes a couple of times a week to thirty minutes every day? Good for you! (In *so* many ways!)

Exercise or Diet for Weight Loss?

I have to make sure you understand just one more concept before we bring this chapter to a close. Exercise is essential for vitality and heart health. You know that. But it isn't necessarily the magic bullet for weight loss.

Some people get very disappointed by how exercise doesn't help them lose that much weight. In fact, you would have to do an extremely large amount of exercise to lose weight without changing a poor diet. If you watch those shows on television where people do extremely intense workouts and lose hundreds of pounds, you may be motivated or you may be intimidated. It certainly doesn't look appealing to me! But those people also have calorie-controlled diets. The exercise helps them build muscle mass, which increases their metabolic rate, meaning they will burn more calories all the time, even when they aren't exercising. But this alone probably will not do the trick if you have a lot of weight to lose.

A few years ago, I was asked to give a talk at a huge health-care conference that included doctors, hospital employees, and staff. The audience included people from all walks of life who work in the health-care industry—nurses, social workers, administrators, secretaries, janitors. I spoke all about exercise and diet and how important exercise was for health and fitness and weight loss. It was my whole "Exercise Is the Best Medication" speech.

There was a doctor speaking after me, and although each speaker only had forty minutes, he spent the first ten minutes of his speech telling the audience (even though this was not the subject of his speech!) that he'd gone on a diet and lost fifty pounds just by changing his diet, and that exercise didn't do a thing.

You could have heard a pin drop. Wasn't he listening to what I had just said? I wanted to put him on a treadmill right then and there, and show him how desperately he actually did need to exercise. No doubt he was completely out of shape with that attitude!

There are so many people waiting for an excuse not to exercise that I wanted to run up and say that we'd planted him there to demonstrate how many people are in denial. There is a theory out there that weight loss is almost all about diet and that exercising just makes you hungrier, so it doesn't really help with weight loss.

But it does help you stay healthy and fit and in a better mood, so you will likely be more motivated to lose weight, and that's a significant benefit. In fact, exercise might even be *more* important than weight loss (although ideally you will accomplish both). Exercise will maintain the tone in your muscles, not only preventing your butt from reaching the floor as you age but also keeping your metabolism up even when you are not exercising. Not only will this help with weight loss, but it may also help with vanity. There's nothing wrong with looking a little more fabulous in your jeans!

Recently there was an article determining whether "fat" or "fit" provided the best cardiovascular protection. This study revealed that if someone was fat but fit, they had less cardiovascular risk than if they were thin and unfit. It also showed that being fit cancelled out some of the risk related to being fat. Exercise really is your best friend, even if you have a bit of a paunch or your pants have been getting noticeably tighter. Don't stop exercising. It is your secret weapon for health.

Here's the bottom line: You *can* lose weight through diet alone, especially if your current diet is poor and very high in fat, carbohydrates, and calories, and you improve it drastically. *However,* the main reason I want you to exercise is for your heart. Yes, exercise burns calories, and that's great, but your cardiovascular fitness is paramount. If your heart isn't working, it doesn't matter how thin and fabulous you are. You have to be fit if you want a healthy heart.

But when you do reach that plateau on your diet (and if you have a lot of weight to lose, you will reach that plateau), don't get frustrated. You've got a secret weapon in your back pocket. You've got exercise. Diet plateaus occur because your metabolism has slowed down, and there is no better way to jump-start your metabolism than with exercise. Losing weight isn't about starving yourself. Some patients, when their weight loss slows down, will suggest the food-withdrawal technique and make the proclamation: "Well, I'll just stop eating."

No, no, no, no, no! Don't stop eating. Start exercising. That's what will help you get to your goal.

Exercise is a topic that people tend to get judgmental about. They quantify it and qualify it. *How many minutes did you do? How fast did you go? What class did you take? What, you don't belong to a gym? Then what do you do?* But at the end of the day, it has nothing to do with any of that. It has to do with fitness. Remember that—it's about getting your heart into condition so it doesn't have to work so hard to perform your normal activities. When you are physically fit, you can exercise, work, take care of your kids, run errands, clean the house, and have fun, and your heart doesn't have to go overboard trying to do it all. It doesn't have to beat so hard. That's fitness. It makes you healthier and it makes you happier, less tired, energized, and feeling better overall.

That's why exercise is the most important thing you can do. It's entirely within your control, so if you do nothing else this book urges you to do, just start exercising most days. Your life will change in wonderful ways.

This Chapter, by Heart

♥ Exercise is the best medication for heart health.

♥ You can calculate your target heart rate and your expected METs level, then give yourself a stress test so you can assess your own fitness level.

♥ Do not give yourself a stress test if you have symptoms or traditional risk factors for heart disease. See your doctor first!

♥ You should be exercising at moderate intensity for 150 minutes every week, or at high intensity for 75 minutes per week. You should also do strength training 2 to 3 days per week.

♥ You don't have to go to the gym. Just move more in your daily life.

♥ Increase your exercise every week or two, so what you are doing is a little bit more difficult than what you were doing the week before.

♥ Start tracking your exercise in your Heart Book, and then get a heart monitor to be sure you are getting your heart rate up enough to enjoy the benefits.

❤ You can lose weight with diet alone, but only exercise will give you cardiovascular fitness, which your heart needs for good health. It can also help you break through weight-loss plateaus.

❤ It is more important to be fit than skinny. Remember that the next time you decide to starve yourself and skip the gym!

PART THREE

All About You

CHAPTER ELEVEN

Let's Get Real

You've got a basic action plan, and now it's time to get personal. In this next section, we're going to talk about why you don't always eat or exercise the way you should, how to take better care of yourself based on your own issues, and how to move forward into a heart-healthier life.

Let's start with the basics. Why aren't you eating right? Why aren't you exercising enough? Even when you *know* you should, when you *know* it's good for you, when you *know exactly what to do* (because you just read Part Two).

I was recently a guest on an early-morning radio show talking about heart health. It was a call-in show, and one after another we received calls from people who, at the crack of dawn, were just getting back from their morning runs. I remember thinking, "Wow, all these amazingly ambitious exercisers!" And then I started to feel guilty. I don't get up at 4:00 a.m. to exercise. I would *never* get up at 5:00 or even 6:00 to exercise. I am lucky if I can drag my half-opened eyes and half-awake self into the shower.

And then I laughed at myself for feeling guilty about something that wouldn't work in my life anyway.

If you are having trouble sticking to the lifestyle you know you should stick to, you are not alone. And you are not lazy. You are not a bad person. You just need to figure out how to make those changes work in your life with your schedule and with your personality. Everyone is different. Everyone has their own clock, their own preferences, their own high and low energy times of day. Exercise doesn't have a clock. Exercise is exercise.

Compliance, or "sticking to it," is one of the most difficult issues to tackle when it comes to changing your lifestyle habits. It isn't that you don't want to improve your health, but somewhere between that desire and practical application, there can be a disconnect. We all *kind of* know what to do (and I hope you know *exactly* what to do if you've read this far), but why is it so hard to do it? Why is it so hard to execute the plan?

I've been thinking about this for a long time. I think part of the problem is one I've already talked about in this book. Public health statistics suggest that this or that exercise is best, or that this or that diet is best, or that this or that time of day is best for that or this. But you are not a statistic. You are an individual, and you might despise morning exercise (high five!) but love an afternoon Zumba class with your friends. You might detest broccoli but happily eat a big salad every day for lunch. You might get impatient with meditation, but yoga makes you feel serene. You are *you*, and once you know what you need to do (as we've discussed in the last two chapters), the only way you are really going to do it is to know yourself well enough to know what you are willing to do.

Lifestyle plans have to accommodate you as the individual, as opposed to you making accommodations for your plans. That may work for a little while, but you will never be able to stick with it, and pretty soon the plan is no longer a plan. It's a former plan, and you're feeling bad about yourself because you think you can't sustain your healthy life program.

It's time we all stop this self-sabotaging, vicious cycle. We only have ourselves, our lives, and our self-love and motivation to propel us forward, so let's give ourselves the best chance we can of being as successful as we can.

In this chapter, I want to help you personalize your plan by getting to know yourself. But don't think you won't have to change a thing. You probably will be inspired to make some changes in your life, changes for your heart, but I want you to do them in a way that is true to who you really are.

This makes me think of a patient who needed to get more exercise. I told her she was going to have a stress test, and to bring in her running shoes. She came in and, somewhat abashedly, showed me what she'd brought in her fashionable tote bag: a pair of kitten heels. "These were the closest thing I could find," she said.

"Really?" I said. "Really? You don't have running shoes?" And so I sat down and wrote her out a prescription for running shoes. I suppose it's no shock that someone who doesn't even own sneakers doesn't exercise. How could she? I've been known to tackle half of Manhattan in four-inch heels, but I wouldn't *exercise* in them . . . at least not on purpose.

When I suggested sneakers, she wrinkled her nose in sheer disgust. Clearly, some old clunky track shoes weren't going to do the trick. I told her to go out and find the cutest, pinkest, sparkliest running shoes she could find. I wanted her to find the sneakers she could love, that made her feel as charming as she feels in those kitten heels, but that would give her that extra oomph to help her want to use them for their intended purpose.

Sometimes you do need to add something to your routine, like more exercise, but if you do, then do it in a way that you enjoy, or we both know it's never going to happen. If I had to go on a treadmill every day, it would never happen. A lot of you probably feel the same way. For me it's simply too boring. When I was in my training and forced myself to go to the gym, I tricked myself this way: I love fashion magazines but would never allow myself to read them, because I knew I had to study. So, whenever I would get on the elliptical trainer for thirty minutes, I would allow myself to read the latest *Glamour*, *Cosmo*, *Allure*, or *Vogue*. It was happy bliss for me. Sweating to my favorite fashions worked for me. It made me look forward to my exercise. I had a magazine budget, just to make sure I could get all the new issues as soon as they came in. This trick helped my own compliance at a time when it sometimes felt easier to just go home and go to bed.

There are multiple diet books out there, and pages and pages of advice about how to modify your behavior. Changing behavior in itself has become a science, and we know that there are stages of behavior change that work. The American Heart Association has studied behavior change and come up with the basic stages that can help effect real behavior change. They are:

1. Pre-contemplation, or thinking about thinking about change
2. Contemplation, or thinking about change
3. Preparation, or actually taking steps to get ready for change
4. Action, or changing
5. Maintenance, or continuing the change

When analyzing these stages, however, I've found that there is a stage missing from this list. Behind the closed doors of my office, I have seen many different types of people. There are those who are scared, others who are in denial, others who are motivated, and some who want to get healthy but just have no idea how to do it. There are the chronic dieters who are still overweight, the yo-yo dieters who have given up, the obsessively food restrictive dieters, and the ones who think they are healthy but really have no idea how badly they eat. Some people are successful at taking control of their lives to get healthy, and others find the process significantly more challenging, but when they aren't able to keep up with lifestyle changes, there are many different reasons. When you read statements like "Achieve and maintain a normal weight," "Exercise more," "Eat more fruits and vegetables," and "Manage stress," you might want to just roll your eyes, but the reason why is unique to *you*. So where is the aspect of individuation in that five-item list? We know that behavior change is critical to lifestyle management, especially if you are at risk for heart disease. We know how important it is to adopt healthy behaviors. What we haven't completely aced is how to make that happen for *everyone*.

Doctors know that just telling patients to do these things isn't enough. There has been a 70 percent increase in obesity in the past decade, an increase in heart attacks in women between the ages of 35 and 55, and an increase in diabetes in all age groups, and the evidence points to lifestyle-based Heart Throbs as responsible for those changing numbers.

The public health system is trying to get the message out, the doctors are trying to tell their patients, and people know that a healthy diet and exercise is crucial. It's not that the message hasn't been received. The buck stops with you! The reality of compliance is about knowing your own human nature and how you function as an individual in order to understand how you can best maintain a lifestyle plan. I'm here to help.

There are multiple different personality tests that have helped people find their most compatible jobs or their most compatible mates, so with that in mind, I've created a personality test, based on thousands of patients I've treated and the behavioral trends I've witnessed, to help you figure out who you are in terms of your ability to stick with the healthy lifestyle choices we talk about in this book. If you understand what lifestyle choices will more likely lead to success and which are more likely to lead to failure, then you can make lifestyle decisions that make sense for you.

The following test will help you to discover your personality type when it comes to diet, exercising, stress reduction, and life balance. Find yourself in these personality types so it will be easier for you to know your potential downfalls. As with all personality types, sometimes you will fit into more than one category, and that's fine. Just read the advice for both types that seem to apply to you. When you realize who you are and where your faults lie, you are more likely to prepare yourself, take a different approach, and prevent disaster. Thanks to all my patients for your trial and error, missteps and mishaps. I've learned so much from you!

Your Diet Style

When it comes to lifestyle, diet often seems to get the most attention. Everyone is trying to figure out the next quick fix, big thing, or plan to make them skinny and svelte without trying too hard. I have unfortunate news for you. No matter what diet you go on, you have to try, and you have to be conscious of what you are eating. Once you accept that, it will help things along.

My patient Phyllis, a 56-year-old woman and a self-described "happy person," has a great job, a great husband, and is enjoying her fifties. She was thirty pounds above her normal weight and her cholesterol and blood pressure were elevated. I suggested it was time to take a closer look at a diet to help her lose weight and manage those two major issues.

She started a Heart Book, and we got a much clearer idea of her habits. We realized that desserts were part of her dinners, and she grabbed a quick and easy bagel from the corner deli a bit too often.

We changed around her meal plan, and I asked that she keep track of it. Upon her next visit, I was in shock. She had gained five pounds. I looked at her Heart Book and realized what had happened. According to her, she was being "so good," eating multigrains and egg whites for breakfast, a salad for lunch, and grilled fish with greens for dinner. Then there was a friend's birthday party, and after having a hamburger on a roll at the barbecue, potato chips, and a piece of cake and ice cream, she figured she'd messed up everything. So the next day, she had a bagel for breakfast, a chocolate chip cookie for a snack, and pizza for lunch. When I saw the lasagna with meat sauce for dinner that same day, I asked her what she was thinking! She said that she messed up, and that it just wasn't worth continuing, so she binged a bit. She would "get back to it."

This is one type of dieter I often see in my office. They mess up and think they can't go right back. They don't see that every minute of life is another opportunity to make a right choice or a wrong choice. If you make a wrong choice, it doesn't mean total destruction. Look for yourself in the questions below and see where you fit in the best. Maybe if you are the all-or-nothing type, you can relate to Phyllis and this advice might help you be more successful with your choices. Or, if you are in denial, it might be important to look in the mirror, get back to that Heart Book, and see who you really are.

Let's get started.

Pick one answer that best describes your diet or the way you tend to eat most of the time:

1. I am all or nothing. Either I do a diet all the way or I don't do it at all.

2. Change scares me. I usually eat the same things, and when I have to change something, it makes me uncomfortable and I change very slowly.

3. I need to be in control and make choices about everything I do. Don't tell me what to eat!

4. If I understand something and it makes sense, then I can do it, but don't give me any mumbo-jumbo. I am rational.

5. My diet is really not that bad. I don't eat much, I eat healthy foods, and I really can't understand why I am overweight.

Depending on your answer, this is your Diet Type:

1. **The Restrictor.** When going on a diet, you need to cut out all offending agents completely. Keep a diet diary for one week to see where you are going wrong, then banish the bad stuff. Go cold turkey. If anybody can do it, you can.

2. **The Reducer.** No meat? No sugar? No, thanks. You are set in your ways, so the best way for you to make changes is to make small slow changes and work to reduce your less healthful choices a little at a time on a regular schedule that makes you comfortable. For example, if you eat a lot of meat, try going meatless on Mondays, and see how that goes. Don't make another change until this one becomes a comfortable habit.

3. **The Minimizer.** You do better counting calories or points rather than having a specific food plan that tells you what to eat. You can make excellent use of a diet diary because all the actual food choice decisions are in your own hands. See what you like to eat, then just minimize your calories or points.

4. **The Rationalist.** You are fine with the "what," as long as you know the "why." For you the key is education. You aren't going to blindly accept anyone's recommendations for anything without knowing the facts, so do your research! Be your own fact-

checker. Reread the heart anatomy chapter in this book, and decide for yourself what you need to do. Then you won't have any trouble doing it.

5. **The Denier.** If you have an overweight issue, you cannot be undereating. You are likely either consuming more food than you think or making less healthy choices than you think, or both. A diet diary will help you see this. You might also benefit from seeing a nutritionist, who can point out where you are going wrong if you can't see it. Somewhere along the line, you are fooling yourself, so it's time to investigate exactly how. When you know where you are likely to go astray, you can choose a dietary program or lifestyle changes that subvert your weakness, whether that means keeping a food diary to keep yourself honest or letting yourself off the hook because you know you will *never* keep up with a food diary but are likely to follow a diet plan. Do some research if you need more information, cut out certain foods for good if that's you, or eat what you want but cut back on portion sizes if that's more your style. Whatever you do, just start making the changes. There are many, many ways to improve your diet. Find the ones that work for *you.*

Your Exercise Style

Alena was determined to get back into shape, so every day on the way to work in the morning, she promised herself she would go to the gym right after work. She was genuinely determined, so much so that she carried with her a little gym bag with her exercise clothes and sneakers. She promised herself optimistically that today was the day to start exercise. But on Monday there was an emergency meeting. On Tuesday there were drinks with friends. On Wednesday she decided to work a little late. On Thursday she was too tired. And on Friday she figured, "Why bother?" She wasn't motivated anymore. Life obviously was too busy.

I hear this story over and over again. I know. I really know. It is not easy fitting it all into one twenty-four-hour period. We are *tired*, and even though we might know, theoretically, that exercise will give us more energy, in the moment it just feels too difficult.

There are so many of us who feel this way that it's easy to justify, and daunting to even know how to start. Is that you? Are you that kind of person who won't do what's not on the schedule? Are you the one who needs to be accountable to a class, a friend, or a time before you'll even consider it? If you can find these qualities in your noncompliance, then the answer is easy. Put it in the schedule and just make it happen. Become accountable to that the same way you would if it were a meeting, or a dinner, or a work obligation.

There are other reasons people fall off the exercise program. See if you can find your issues in the questions below, then let's understand what you can do about it to ensure success. Success isn't difficult; it just has to make sense to you and who you are.

Pick one answer that best describes your typical approach to exercise:

1. If I am going to do something, I sign up 150 percent. I am not afraid to do it.

2. If I'm going to be successful at something, I can't be obsessed. It needs to fit into my life.

3. If it is planned, I will do it. Just put it in the schedule.

4. I get bored so easily. It is hard for me to focus on one thing for very long.

5. I might not get sweaty, but I am very active and I do enough.

How social are you when it comes to exercise?

1. I like to exercise alone.

2. I like to exercise in a group.

When do you have the most energy?

1. Rise and shine. I am a morning person.

2. I can stay up all night long; just don't wake me in the morning.

Depending on your answers, this is your Exercise Type:

1. **The Obsessor**. You need a routine that will keep you exercising after the initial thrill wears off, and you also have to guard against overdoing it at first and injuring yourself. You do best with a structured program, like an intense group class or team where they will notice when you don't show up or when training for a goal, like a 5K. You are goal-oriented and you like to meet your goals. You also like intensive exercise like aerobics, with an edge of competition like sports.

2. **The Minimalist**. You don't like your exercise experience to be intense, but you will benefit if you keep it very regular. Look for exercises you enjoy that you can fit into your normal routine, like walking around a track every morning or hitting the treadmill at the gym every day after work before you go home. You don't have to exhaust yourself. Just take it easy until you feel like doing more. It's better to do something than to do nothing. Changing your routine can be difficult at first, but just keep reminding yourself that once it becomes a habit, it will feel like you've always done it, and your health will benefit greatly.

3. **The Scheduler.** Join a gym and put your sessions on the calendar, sign up for a class and put it on your schedule, or block out time for your walk or run along a planned course. You are busy and you do best with exercise that has a scheduled beginning and end time, like a class or particular running route that you know takes X number of minutes. If you have a trainer who is waiting for you, chances are you will show up on time and do the work. If you don't want to hire a trainer, then commit to working out with a friend and meeting her there.

4. **The Variety Lover.** Variety Lovers get bored easily, so they absolutely need to mix things up if they are going to make exercise a regular part of their lives. Find something for all your different sides—yoga on Mondays, weightlifting on Tuesdays, tennis on Wednesdays. Otherwise you know you'll find something more interesting to do.

5. **The Denier.** The American Heart Association says that to be healthy, you need 150 minutes of moderate exercise per week. Just being active may not be enough. Time yourself. You have to know what you are really doing if you want to get healthy. And putting it on your calendar but not actually doing it does not count. You might benefit from a heart monitor so you can actually tell if you are getting your heart rate up. Seeing what you are actually doing rather than what you think you are doing might be crucial to getting the right amount of exercise for you.

Bonus Points:

For each answer above, there is an additional consideration: timing. Consider whether you prefer solitary exercise or group exercise and whether you have the most energy for exercise in the morning or the evening. Then don't schedule activities you know you won't really enjoy because of all the people, or lack of them. Also, plan your exercise for when you know you will have the energy. Stop the self-sabotage. Now that you know what is most suitable for you, go with it. You might be able to stick with it more easily than you thought.

Your Stress Management Style

I've said it before, and I will say it again: Everyone has stress. Every single person I have ever met has some kind of stress. But, like beauty, stress is in the eye of the beholder. Some people are stressed if their routines are broken, they can't find their favorite brand of something, or the woman who regularly cuts their hair moved and didn't tell them (yes, I had someone tell me this was one of her greatest stressors!). For some it is paying the rent, covering the cost of all the bills, managing their aging parents without help, or being a good mother. Regardless of the gravity of each of these situations, the self-perceived amount of stress is what is critical.

Then I see those women who are juggling it all—family, work, kids, parents, and their own illness. Sometimes they will shed a tear or two in my office, but then they stop and keep moving forward. They have friends to rely on, and they know that they have no choice but to move forward.

I want you to understand that your stress is *your* stress, and only you can judge it or decide how much it will affect you. Get the best perspective on it that you can, knowing that you can't compare your story or your reality to anyone else's, but understand what it means in the big picture of your life. Then understand that you have to manage it and figure out a way that the stress hormones won't keep running through your body, wreaking havoc on your endothelium, arteries, blood pressure, and every other organ system. Know that you need to figure out how to get those stress hormones under control, because if you don't, it can make you sick.

Stress is okay. Stress is normal. It's how you manage it that matters.

Pick one answer that best describes your typical approach to stress management:

1. I can handle anything. Why do I need stress management?

2. If I have to focus on dealing with my stress, I guess I can try, but just thinking about it is stressing me out. Is it really worth it?

3. I'm overwhelmed. Just tell me what to do, and I'll do it. I don't want to have to come up with something on my own. That's asking too much.

4. If I could fit in some kind of stress management, then I would. I would love to be able to take that time for myself, but I just don't have room in my schedule and it seems like a luxury.

5. Everyone has stress. What am I going to do about it? It's normal.

Depending on your answers, this is your Stress Management Type:

1. **The Deliberator.** You don't think you need help. In fact, you thrive on stress. However, you are taxing your adrenal glands, and that constant flow of stress hormones through your bloodstream is wreaking havoc on your body. You need to understand and recognize when stress is helping you and when it's hurting you. Even if you feel okay, start paying attention to your stress and force yourself to spend a little time relaxing every day, even if you are just singing your theme song (more details to follow on page 271). Notice how you feel as you relax, your blood pressure goes down, and your heart rate slows. The more

you practice this, the more your body will learn to counteract the effects of chronic stress. And consider breathing as part of your day. Ten deep inhalations for a count of six and exhalations for a count of four. That might be all you need.

2. **The Doser.** If you are too stressed to even think about stress management, then you need to give yourself a daily dose of stress relief. Try starting your day with a five-minute relaxation exercise, and then do it again in the late afternoon. Even something as simple as ten deep breaths, inhaling to the count of six and exhaling to the count of four, can have a wonderful stress-relieving effect on your body, and you can certainly spare five minutes to do this. Or deliberately close your eyes and be still, either sitting in a chair or lying down, door closed, phone off. Do it for five minutes, then ten minutes, twice a day. Shut your mind off and focus on your breathing, or the weight of your feet on the ground, or your body on the floor. Focus on you and no other information. This is the time to listen to your heartbeat instead of the chatter in your mind.

3. **The Quantifier**. You need to find someone to help you manage your stress. We all need help sometimes, so why not get the help you need? Many good therapists are qualified to teach you stress management techniques. Or try a meditation or yoga class. Or just talk to a friend who seems to be good at managing stress and see if you can get some action strategies you can try every day. Then follow through and do it. It will make a big difference. Help sometimes is a necessity. Just as you might need a medication if you have a heart problem, get professional assistance if you need it. Being taught to meditate or do Reiki could benefit you for a lifetime, so consider learning from a professional, so you can carry it with you for the rest of your life and use it.

4. **The Pragmatist**. You think stress management is a luxury, but it's actually a therapy, and you need to think about it this way so you can justify the time it takes. Then fit it in the schedule and honor your appointments as seriously as you would honor your dental or doctor appointments. Yoga, biofeedback, or even a scheduled evening bath or regular massage can start to feel as necessary as they actually are once you make them a priority.

5. **The Denier**. Yes, everyone has stress some of the time, but if you feel stressed every day, that is definitely not normal, even if it is all too common these days. If everyone else was jumping off a bridge, would you do it? Wait, don't answer that! Instead, just do what the doctor says and do something about it. Even if you sit quietly for a few minutes every day with your eyes closed practicing deep breathing, you will start to realize the benefits. Then you'll learn what normal is really supposed to feel like.

Whatever your style, it's time to tackle your stress—a little at a time, here and there, in ways you enjoy. That's the key—if you don't enjoy it, you will just get more stressed. Let yourself relax doing something you love in a way that works for you and your heart will relax too.

Your Pleasure Style: How You Enjoy Your Life

This is a tough one, especially following the stress section. Believe it or not, laughing and smiling and enjoying life are crucial to heart health and should never be considered an extra benefit, even if things get too busy. You need to make time to have fun, nurture your spirit, and do something that puts a smile on your face.

Renee has a job in real estate and is married with three kids. She is juggling a lot between caring for her children and being the major breadwinner in her family. She is always running somewhere to meet with clients or picking up one of her kids. I asked her what she did for fun. She looked at me like I was crazy.

I explained the importance of laughing and smiling and enjoying her life, and she explained that there was no time for that. Things might slow down for her somewhere around 11:00 p.m., she said, but by then she was ready for bed, not laughing. I understood the sarcasm, but I persisted, explaining the data on the benefits of joy and laughter in health and wellness and life satisfaction. I asked her what she enjoyed. She said that in college she used to knit, and she actually really liked it. She stopped knitting when she didn't have the time or the patience anymore after she started having children. When we even broached the subject about how to incorporate this little bit of joy into her life every day, she actually got excited and decided to stop by her old yarn shop to see what they had. She'd never even considered that she might be able to fit this one small thing for herself back into her schedule, and once she'd discovered the possibility, a light went on inside of her. She just needed permission.

I am hereby giving you permission to have fun! Whatever you do for fun doesn't have to be a sweeping gesture of craziness fun. It just needs to be something that provides you with a little bit of happiness. Is it reading a book? Going to the movies? Hanging out with friends? Bungee jumping or snow skiing? Is it training for a triathlon or running a seven-minute mile, like you used to do in college?

Find your own joy. Look into that part of your spirit that you might have left behind as your life got more complicated and stressful. Find out what can give you joy and make you happy. Plan for it and look forward to it, and then *do it*! In the meantime, be with your friends, laugh with your family, and open your heart and your soul to the joy that you can find in life. Remind yourself, whenever you are tempted to cancel your "fun" plans, how important they are. The benefits will be beyond what you expect. There is nothing like having a truly happy heart filled with joy.

Pick one answer that best describes how you view joy, fun, and pleasure in your life—things that are crucial for living from the heart:

1. I have to love something in order to do it, and to love it, it had better be fast, hard, or give me a rush. Hanging out on the beach isn't for me.

2. I love to do things when I know I'll be able to see the end result. "Fun" in itself isn't enough.

3. Being with people is the best place I can be, especially family or friends. To me that's the ultimate pleasure.

4. Give me a book and a quiet corner on the couch and I couldn't be happier.

5. I have joy every night when I watch reality TV. Those people are so ridiculous, it cracks me up.

Depending on your answers, this is your Pleasure Style:

1. **The Passion Player.** You passionate types need to do things that are thrilling or exciting. Take some risks and be daring to really fulfill your naturally adventurous side. Otherwise you'll get bored, and boring is no fun, right?

2. **The Processor.** The process type enjoys creating and making things most of all. An arts and crafts project or crocheting a sweater would be ideal choices. To you true pleasure comes from saying, "See what I did?" or "This is what I made!"

3. **The Lover.** Lovers thrive on being around friends and family and are happiest surrounded by people they love. Schedule regular dinner parties, family gatherings, or just big gabfests with family or friends for true fulfillment.

4. **The Individualist.** The individualist gets rest, replenishment, and true pleasure by taking a break from social interaction. Prioritize your downtime. You need it! Find time to be alone, to relax, and to do something you really enjoy. Tell the massage therapist you'd rather not talk.

5. **The Denier.** What, you're here in this category again? Girl, you need to spend some time looking in the mirror! It's so important to have fun in life, but staring at a television and mocking other people's lives, while entertaining, isn't what I mean by pleasure, not to mention joy or fun. Instead, get out there. Go to a funny play or a comedy club. Laugh with your most hilarious friends. Let your sense of humor engage with the real world rather than with a television screen. You'll be a better woman for it.

Once you understand your tendencies, your preferences, and your individual style, you will greatly increase your chances of sticking to a self-care plan that includes a healthy diet, regular exercise, and stress management. You are worth an investment in these crucial lifestyle changes, so spend time getting to know yourself well enough to know that while you may not be up running five miles at 4:30 a.m., you do know for a fact that after work you will be in yoga class, and then you're going out with the girls.

Because that's *fun.* This can be your new life. You're going to love it because you're finally going to feel good enough to truly enjoy it! It just takes a little bit of getting to know yourself. Welcome to *you.* Start now doing what you can. A little change here, a little change there. Learn your personal style and needs, because one size does not fit all, and then change a little more. And a little more. Until one day you wake up healthy, fit, relaxed, and *happier*.

This Chapter, by Heart

♥ Lifestyle changes don't work the same for everyone. It's not enough to want to change or to know what to do. You also have to figure out how to change in a way that is realistic for you.

♥ If you understand the realities of your lifestyle and your personality, you will be better able to implement lifestyle changes you can stick to. For example, you may not be the person who can exercise at 4:00 a.m., but you might be the person who can exercise at 7:00 p.m.

♥ Learn your diet, exercise, stress management, and pleasure styles in order to stay motivated and enjoy your new heart-healthy lifestyle.

CHAPTER TWELVE

Health Care Is Self-Care

There is more to a healthy life than diet and exercise. You already know that, but are you living it? Let's get you on track by covering some of the other important aspects of your life, especially the four S's: stress, sex, sleep, and supplements. Each of these areas can have a profound positive or negative affect on your health, your sense of well-being, and your heart.

Women tend to put themselves last, and that contributes to dysfunction in the four S's: We get stressed, we stop having sex, we don't sleep well, and we forget to keep an eye on our nutrient intake, including supplements that could help us do all those previous S-words better.

I'm not going to say that taking care of yourself is simple. The truth is, sometimes it isn't easy at all. In fact, if it were easy to do the right things for ourselves all the time, we wouldn't gain too much weight, get out of shape, get involved in the wrong relationships, or let stress get the better of us. Taking care of yourself big picture is hard, but here's the truth: Taking care of yourself little picture isn't so hard after all. It's in our nature to care for others, but when we break down, everybody else is out of luck, aren't they? So let *you* be on your list of people you are so committed to caring about, and just watch what you can accomplish.

Of course, that all sounds nice, but you may already be thinking: Who has the time? We just don't have the time to take care of ourselves, or so we tell ourselves. Trust me, I know. But the fact is that self-care will add minutes to your day because it promotes habits that give you more energy and relieves stress that makes you unproductive. Self-care is about what you eat and how you exercise, but it's also about how you take care of the rest of you—your emotions, your relationships, even the joy you take in life and the way you treat yourself when you get sick.

So how do we practice true self-care on a daily basis, when the schedule, the clock, and the many demands of our crazy lives dictate that there are other "more important" things to do?

Heart Sense

I have an extremely busy life, as you can imagine! The key to "doing it all" is staying organized. I plan my life by the weeks, making my checklists, but no matter what else is going on, I have a date with myself I never break. I get my nails done. I get them painted red.

This is my personal self-care ritual. My manicurist, Aurora, is a kind and nurturing soul. (A few of her recipes are in the back of this book.) She comes in early or stays late for me if necessary, and every week we have this date, full of girl talk. It makes me feel girly and pretty and taken care of, and all of those feelings in the middle of the craziness make a big difference for me. It's my thing.

Without it, I could not be as grounded and as centered as I am.

I'm not telling you to go get your nails done. I'm sure you have your own thing—the thing that would make you feel grounded and centered. If you don't, find it! Write about it in your Heart Book until you figure out what it should be. Make a date with yourself that you keep every week, no matter what. This is how you get to know yourself better. If you never spend any time with yourself, how will you know who you are, and who you are becoming?

Trust me, it is worth it.

De-stress by Taking Your Life Back

First, let's talk about stress. I've already mentioned stress quite a bit in this book, but that's only because it's so incredibly important. You know it's a heart disease risk, but let's look more closely at how you can take care of yourself by reducing your stress. When you feel like you've lost control of the wheel and your life is spinning like a car out of control, you can stop the spinning. There are ways to regain control.

My patient Jennifer came in once every four months for palpitations and chest pain. At 46 years old, she was diagnosed with high blood pressure, and she was upset about having to be on medication and frustrated with her whole life. She was so stressed out that I felt the room vibrate with her nervous energy as she rapid-fire explained to me her job stress, kid stress, husband drama, and family pain. She was having stress on every level, with her parents sick and living across the country, her siblings not participating in her parents' care, and her commute to her new job that she hated but took anyway because of the financial struggles after her husband lost his job. Her kids, 10 and 7, needed to be in two different places at the same time,

and she didn't know how to get them there with the job and the commute and the parents and with her husband interviewing for new
employment. Every time she told me what was going on in her life, I
had palpitations too! Who could blame her for being so stressed?

But stress was taking its toll. She wasn't sleeping, she was bum-
ming cigarettes off friends, and she was constantly munching on
baked potato chips (she thought they were healthier than the regular
ones until I reminded her of her *blood pressure* and the salt content!).
I knew she needed to start her own Heart Book so she could figure
out the windows of time when she could take control and take her
life back.

We started with her commute. As we chatted, it came out that she
really missed being up on the latest bestselling trashy novels that she
and her friends would swap and chat about. We realized she could
take the train to work instead of driving her car. She could relax and
read all the way to work. Voilà—Jennifer time! We also found another mother whose children were in the same activities as Jennifer's
and who was willing to lend a helping hand with the chauffeuring.
And she found a babysitter to help out two days a week so after work
she could go to yoga class.

This is how Jennifer grabbed the steering wheel of her life, and
the domino effect of taking control of her health and providing herself with some self-care changed her life. Six months later, she still
had stressors, but they weren't *stressing* her the way they were before.
Her life felt much better to her.

You can do this too. Break down your life and find those pockets
of time you can reserve just for you. This isn't just a nice thing to
do—it is absolutely essential. Every one of us has within us the spirit
to become that ideal vision of ourselves, but when we wake up in the
morning and think that we just can't do it for one more day, that
spirit can seem far away and unfamiliar. This is the time to really take

a look at what *you* need. Put away the "buts" for a second. You know what I mean. ("I would go to the gym, *but* . . ." or "I used to love to take yoga classes, *but* . . ." or "I'd eat less junk food, *but* . . .") Let's start with what you can control. Do it because you have to—because one day you will get sick if you don't.

This attitude shift is key, so let's look at how you can change your mind to change your stress, and thereby change your life. It's all about mastering the art of well-being.

Your Theme Song

I strongly suggest to all my patients that they have a theme song. A theme song is a song that expresses how you feel, or how you want to feel, during stressful situations. Sing it to yourself and you gain courage, motivation, and a better attitude. I think there are times I couldn't have survived without my theme song. During some of the hardest times of my life, I found a song that fit my life's current theme and gave me a little push forward.

A theme song is not only inspiration; it also plays a little trick on you. When you sing it out loud, or even under your breath, you actually have to *breathe*. You can't hold your breath or hyperventilate if you are singing. This is a great way to keep your heart rate down, blood pressure low, and even stop a panic attack in its tracks.

I have a couple of theme songs I've used throughout my life. I've had a theme song for many of those phases in life when it was tough or I felt anxious. My standard fallback always seems to be "The Greatest Love of All" by Whitney Houston. When things get stressful, when I have a big meeting, before a talk, or when I'm headed onto a television set, I have been known to sing it under my breath, just to give me that extra boost of confidence. It actually helps to remember that the greatest love of all is inside of me! I sing it like I mean it—because I do mean it!

Find your song by remembering a time when you felt empowered, strong, or happy. Envision yourself in the movie of your life, and sing your song to yourself. Let it help you take control, de-stress, get grounded, and, of course, breathe.

Mastering the Art of Well-Being

One of the most effective ways to deal with stress is to adjust your attitude. Although there is some evidence that some people have a natural tendency to be more positive than others, anybody can choose to see a situation from any direction. When you decide that you are important, that you are worth taking care of, and that part of your day will always be devoted to *you*, your stress level will begin to drop.

This is how you master the art of well-being. To live a heart-centered life means to get up every morning knowing how important it is that you don't just check off everything on your list but that you move through your life knowing who you are, taking charge of your day, and making the conscious decision, over and over again, to take care of yourself *before* you take care of anybody else. In the medical literature, they call this self-nurturance. Self-nurturance means engaging yourself in activities that nourish you. Whether that means going for a five-mile run or putting bubble bath in the bathtub and lighting candles or putting aside time to write your novel or start your own business is your call. Your doctor isn't going to tell you to do it, but it is important, because this is what lifts the burden of stress from your shoulders.

Another part of this is knowledge, including the knowledge you are gaining about your heart, your Heart Throbs, and how you are living. Women with greater knowledge of their Heart Throbs and cardiovascular disease are more likely to practice self-nurturance. Those women who didn't know about their Heart Throbs were less likely to take care of themselves and were more likely to have more stress as well as less financial stability and less of a feeling of control over their lives in general.

But this is about more than knowledge—it's about how knowledge can influence your *perception*. For example, when you find work that you are passionate about, even if you work twelve-hour days, it's not stressful. Finding what you love to do is an important way to take control of your life. Doing what makes you happy keeps stress at bay, because the focus is not on the stress anymore. It's on your happiness.

A recent study from the Harvard School of Public Health just came out, and it's all over the news as I write this. It's one of the first large studies to ever look at the effects of *positive* emotional states specifically on heart health.

We've known for many years that negative emotional states like depression, anxiety, hostility, and pessimism can hurt the heart. This study flipped the switch, looking at what actually had a positive influence on the heart, because the absence of a Heart Throb isn't the same thing as the presence of a positive influence. The results are so exciting, because the study supports exactly what I've witnessed over many years and exactly what I tell my patients: There is a clear link between positive emotional states and a healthier heart.

People who are the most optimistic have a 50 percent reduced risk of experiencing a first heart attack. Also linked with decreased heart disease were an overall sense of well-being, life satisfaction, and happiness. It's not just about getting rid of the Heart Throbs. It's about living from the heart, with joy and purpose, with self-love and personal satisfaction. Those things keep the heart strong and healthy, or they help it to heal much faster than it would heal without them.

I believe this is critical for doctors to understand: that "prescribing" a glass-half-full approach to life may be just as important as prescribing a daily dose of aspirin! But it's even more critical for *you* to understand, because you are the only one who can change the way you think about things. You are the only one who knows your own mind. Your doctor can't turn you into an optimist. Your doctor can't prescribe life satisfaction, fulfilling work, purpose, joy, vitality, and happiness.

Can you become an optimist, even if you tend toward the pessimistic? Can you find life satisfaction if you don't feel like you have it right now? Can you acquire self-love, like you might acquire a new pair of shoes?

Yes, yes, yes!

One way is to have more fun. Laugh more. Let yourself feel more pleasure. Joy and laughter and fun don't just make your life more enjoyable. They actually make your heart healthier. An Oxford University study showed that laughter improves immune function, lowers blood pressure, enhances mood, and decreases stress and depression.

Another study compared people who watched the very serious and intense movie *Saving Private Ryan* with people who watched funny movies like *There's Something About Mary* and *Shallow Hal.* The *Private Ryan* viewers had blood vessels that constricted 30 to 50 percent, but those watching the funny movies had blood vessels that dilated. The beneficial effects of laughing for just ten to fifteen minutes can last for twenty-four hours!

States like optimism and happiness and joy might seem like they are easier for some people than others, but even if you don't think of yourself as the naturally cheerful type, know that optimism and a positive attitude are learned behaviors, just like pessimism and a negative attitude. If you can stop biting your nails, if you can remember to brush your teeth every day, then you can stop a bad habit and you can start a good one.

It all comes down to control. When you decide that you are in control of your attitude and the way you see your life, then your life will begin to change. You can be a victim of your circumstances or you can seek out purpose and meaning. As doctors, we know that people with a more positive attitude do better, get less sick, and are less likely to suffer, even if we don't know or can't exactly prove why. I see every day how much of an impact a patient's attitude has on her health habits as well as how well she recovers from a health problem. The role of victim may seem like the natural place to go when something bad happens to you, but the real empowerment comes not in wondering, "Why me?" but in thinking, "So what am I going to do about it now?"

The patients who believe that they can try harder, compared to those who feel defeated before they even begin, do much better overall. So let's make this your new attitude. Let's empower you to flip the switch.

Flipping the switch is about understanding that you really can change your life. So shut it down. Turn it off. Change the channel. Try it. It feels really good. And if you mess up, don't worry. If you lapse into anxiety or pessimism or depression, remind yourself that this is a process, and every minute of life means you have another chance to do something differently or better. Every day is a brand-new one, just like Spencer said. You can keep starting all over again.

There is always good. It's in your heart.

Get Sexy

I know you've been waiting for this part, haven't you? Yes, it's time to talk about sex. Now, don't get embarrassed! Why shouldn't we talk about this? Girlfriend to girlfriend? Because sex is important. The American Heart Association says so!

It's true. In January 2012, the American Heart Association released its first-ever scientific statement related to sexual activity, and I love that they said, "Sexual activity is important for quality of life." They also said that "impaired sexual activity is often associated with anxiety, depression, and other psychosocial factors."

So let's talk about sex. It's important. I'd even say it's vital. If the American Heart Association can do it, so can we!

I've seen the gamut—women who think they aren't supposed to talk about sex, women who think they aren't even supposed to like it, and women who (like a woman I met recently who owns her own sex toy company) will speak quite freely and openly about how masturbation with sex toys changed their lives. (I tried not to be embarrassed, sitting there next to her on a panel discussion in my proper business suit!)

But here's the fact: We are sexual beings, whether we are comfortable talking about it or not. We are biologically programmed to want and need sex, and for most people, a healthy sex life is a sign of overall health. When things go wrong in that department, it's usually a sign that things are going wrong elsewhere. It's a measure of vitality, no less than a stress test or resting heart rate are.

So whether it gets you excited or makes you uncomfortable, let's talk about sex, and I'll tell you what I know.

I think that when *Sex and the City* came on television, it really changed the landscape of how women communicate about sex. Suddenly, right there in plain view, we could watch women talking about wanting to have sex. For many women this was a revelation. The character of Samantha, in particular, broke down barriers about sexual communication, but every one of those women was a sort of female archetype—the creative one who was seeking true love, the prim and proper one who was concerned about what society thought of her, the self-made power woman who was devoted to her career, and of course, Samantha, the one who saw sex as her favorite hobby. We could all relate to at least one of these types, and it opened a discussion that I believe has really helped a lot of women.

But we still don't tend to talk about sex with our doctors. We talk about sex with our girlfriends (or we should, when appropriate), but doctors? Especially male doctors? Embarrassing, right? So we don't ask the questions we really want to ask. You may not even be sure your doctor knows the answer. And really, you don't know about his sex life, so why should he know about yours? It's private business, isn't it? Even though it's a fact of life?

A lot of my female patients talk to me about sex, but I suspect it's because I'm so chatty. My patients and I sometimes slip into girlfriend mode, which seems to make them more comfortable confiding in me. It really helps me learn the true story of their lives, not just the physical stories but all of it, and that allows me to take better care of them because I better understand their big picture.

Oftentimes, it can be hard to get women to confide in their doctors. Men seem to have an easier time with this problem. They may be embarrassed about sexual performance issues, but their doctors tend to ask about them because in men, impotence is a sign of heart disease. It signifies an issue with circulation. More specifically, failure to get an erection can be due to endothelial dysfunction (that arterial lining I keep telling you about) and plaque formation in the arteries. If sufficient blood isn't getting . . . you know . . . *down there* . . . then there might be a problem somewhere along the line. In fact, doctors are quite concerned with impotence, and science has concocted all kinds of drugs to help men with this problem. (Even the ads on television for erectile dysfunction drugs urge men: *Talk to your doctor!*) Impotence can also be a side effect of some medications. Doctors consider male sexual dysfunction to be an *important problem*, and I'm not saying it's not. But my point is that it's just as important in women.

It is time that we talk about sexual dysfunction in women too, as it seems men's penises have gotten all the attention.

Low sexual desire in women isn't specifically a heart risk because it's not directly related to poor circulation like it sometimes can be in men. However, in my opinion, low sexual desire *is* a sign of a heart-related issue. There is a diagnosis called hypoactive sexual desire disorder, meaning the patient has no interest in sex whatsoever. Once upon a time, this was called "being frigid."

When one of my patients has this problem, to me it means that either she is not as healthy as she could be or she is under too much stress, which we know can affect the heart. It could also mean that her interpersonal emotional relationship isn't as healthy as it could be. Personal distress can lead to real-life heart disease, even if the route is more circuitous in women than it can be in men.

Another difference between men and women is that in women, sexual desire does not necessarily precede sexual arousal. In men the desire for sex may come first, and then the sex can lead to the desire to nurture an intimate relationship. In women it's just the opposite. Women want to nurture the relationship, so they go ahead and have sex, even if they don't necessarily feel like it. Once they get started, they're often glad they did it. A lot of women feel like this and don't realize how common it is. They think something is wrong with them because the desire for sex itself isn't primary, but we can't all be Samantha. I am not saying to do something you don't want to do, but just know that studies have shown that if you do it, you just might be glad that you did.

Your body will be glad too. One of the reasons sex is so healthy for you is that it releases oxytocin, which makes you feel good and closely bonded with your partner. It also releases anti-inflammatories, hormonal painkillers, and immunoglobulins, which can help boost the immune system, so it can actually have a healing effect on your body. In addition to all that good stuff, sex also releases other feel-good hormones like endorphins, so sex is a little dose of happy medicine.

And then you've got the emotional effect. When you are having regular sex in your thirties, forties, fifties, sixties, or beyond, you are more likely having it within the context of a loving relationship than you were in your twenties, when you still might have been searching for the right partner. Sex is a way to connect with your significant other in a way you don't connect with anybody else. There is something about the routine of maintaining intimacy that forges a connection beyond words. It's hormonal as well as emotional.

You don't even have to have actual sex to get the benefits of a healthy sex life. Men and women in their eighties reported being satisfied with their sex lives, even if that meant just hugging and holding hands. Humans have a deep need for physical contact. Many studies have demonstrated the importance of physical touch for emotional well-being as well as for health. It begins with babies and extends throughout life. Physical touch triggers hormone release, and those hormones benefit your health and mood. You can't get these benefits from a vitamin. You can't find them in a health food store (unless you hug the cashier!). Everybody is always looking for a quick fix, so here is yours: Eat right, exercise, and have sex.

Safe Sex

A study came out just this year from the American College of Cardiology that tracked people who had already had a heart attack, and it asked them whether anyone had discussed sexual activity with them upon discharge from the hospital. Forty-seven percent of men had received information about the safety of sexual activity, but only 30 percent of women had received this information.

Among those who didn't receive any information about sexual activity post–heart attack, most of them were *not* having sex a year after discharge—both men and women. They were afraid to try. A lot of my patients who have heart disease wonder if sex is safe. Even those without heart disease but who are out of shape wonder if sex will put too much of a strain on their hearts. The American Heart Association has actually weighed in on this issue! They state that if you can walk up two flights of stairs, then it is safe to have sex. The risk of a heart attack during sex is quite low. So there's your test. Can you walk up two flights of stairs? If yes, then go ahead and get it on.

Healthy Sex at Any Age

Something very interesting happens with the sex drive as women go through perimenopause and menopause. There is a perception that as women get older, they don't want to have sex, but a study showed that sexual activity in older women is actually associated with good health and with being in a loving relationship and with a healthy emotional connection to another person. Impressively, 10 percent of the women in the study who were 80 years old or older reported arousal, lubrication, and orgasm.

Healthy sexual activity is also associated with taking hormone replacement therapy (HRT). I had a patient who was taking hormone replacement therapy for a while, but then decided to go off the treatment. When this happened, she noticed a marked decrease in her desire. She told me, "I need my mojo back! I don't feel sexy!" Sex had been a huge part of her life with her husband and it was very important to her. She felt like she'd lost that.

Hormone replacement therapy, and also testosterone supplementation, probably are helpful because they can ease typical menopausal symptoms like vaginal dryness. They can also increase libido, but hormonal therapy is not the only thing that can. Exercise has been shown to have a similar effect. For many women, it keeps the mojo alive. If you are going through a rough time in the sex department, get your heart rate up and start sweating outside the bedroom first. The trickle-down effect may reach your bedroom sooner than you think.

Also, for those who don't want to take HRT orally, I sometimes recommend estrogen suppositories or creams. For some, a simple lubricant is enough to keep them going. But for others, the problem is more than mechanical.

If your sexual activity has dwindled, or you just "don't feel like it" lately, this is a sign from your body that something is out of balance. If you are having health problems, lack of desire could be related to them, but it is also often related to just not feeling good about yourself, not feeling as attractive as you used to feel, not feeling sexy. Do you feel old? You need to get your groove back!

And guess who is most likely to feel like this? In this one study of 50,000 U.S. women ages 18 to 101, low desire and low libido were the most common in women 45 to 64 years old. This age group also reported more sexually related distress issues than in the older or younger woman. That means you're going to feel even better about sex when you are older, so you might as well get started now. You don't have to be a part of this temporary lull. Remind yourself that this is a transitional time in a woman's life, and transitions come with a few bumps in the road. We're under so much stress that sex can begin to feel like just one more thing on your checklist that you have to do. It's not because you're getting older. It's because you're getting *busier* (and not in the good way).

What I really want you to realize is that sexual problems don't exist in a vacuum. They aren't a separate issue from the rest of your life. Sex is part of being human, vital, and alive at every age, from adolescence on. Sex helps you to sustain your sense of self and feel like a woman. It has nothing to do with age—plenty of older women are whoopin' it up at least once or twice a week. Your so-called flaws related to aging are irrelevant too. The person who loves you doesn't care about that. Connection is the key, not a mutual critical assessment of body parts. Just stop doing that to yourself. It isn't kind!

In essence, sex is about the heart, and this is a time of life in which you need to be nurturing your heart, so nurture your heart through sex. Consider it a prescription: Have more sex! And if you simply aren't currently in a relationship where sex is possible or practical? Well, then. (Ahem.) You can *still* enjoy many of the wonderful biochemical benefits of orgasm on your own. The studies all show that there doesn't necessarily need to be another person involved. Keep yourself "tuned up" by giving yourself a little boost of sexual pleasure when you need it, and when someone else does enter your life, if that should happen, you will have maintained that impulse and urge in yourself. And that's all good too.

Sex as Cardio?

Sometimes, when my patients are having heart issues and I want to get more information, I will put a heart monitor on them (I talk more about heart monitors in Chapter 8). One of the first things they often say is, "I am totally going to have sex with this on. Will you be able to tell?" When I get the results of the monitor, we sometimes will look back together and they will point out to me when they were having sex. Sure enough, we will see an increase in heart rate. (By the way, my men patients never do that. As the saying goes, girls will be girls . . .) And just in case you were wondering, the amount of physical effort that shows up on the heart monitor during sex is *never* as much of an increase as with exercise, so despite all its other benefits, sex *does not* count as your cardio. You still have to do that too. Sorry!

Sleep More

Sometimes when you go to bed, you really just want to sleep. And you should sleep. You should probably sleep more, because we are not a nation of healthy sleepers.

Most women barely get six hours per night, so we're already teetering on the edge of risk just by staring at the television for an hour too long at night, trying to wind down (even though television is a stimulant—what are we thinking?).

In a small study called the Pittsburgh Sleep Quality Index, which looked at sleep quality and frequency of sleep symptoms, biomarkers in poor sleepers (defined as those who had trouble falling asleep more than two nights per week, took more than thirty minutes to fall asleep, or woke frequently during the night) were compared to biomarkers in those who slept well. Almost half the people in the study were designated as poor sleepers, and women self-reported more sleep disruption than men.

The people who had the most difficulty falling asleep reported the highest degree of psychological stress. They also had higher fasting insulin levels (indicating prediabetes) and more inflammatory markers. Poor sleep quality has also been associated with greater incidence of being overweight or obese, higher levels of stress hormones, and poorer health habits when you are awake, especially poor eating habits.

That means when you lie in bed with your eyes wide open, going through the checklist for tomorrow, or reviewing the nasty conversation you had with your boss, or worrying about getting the ingredients for the cookies you promised to bake for your daughter's bake sale, you are worse off. Those who take the longest to fall asleep probably are in a mental place of perseveration and self-torture, causing stress hormones to run rampant throughout their bodies, leading to inflammation and obesity.

Several studies have examined how sleep deprivation influences leptin levels in the body. Leptin is the hormone that signals when you are full. When you don't get enough sleep, your leptin levels drop, and you are more likely to overeat because you don't realize when you've had enough. If you are trying to get your weight down to a healthier place, lack of sleep can destroy your resolve. It's biochemical.

Poor sleep can also increase blood pressure. One study looked at a group of men and how much time they spent in slow-wave sleep, the period of deepest sleep. The men with the least amount of time in slow-wave sleep had an 80 percent increased risk of developing high blood pressure over the course of the study. Although there were no women in the study (as is so often the case), it makes sense that we can extrapolate these results to women, and that less slow-wave sleep for us might also increase blood pressure.

For women in particular, poor sleep quality was not only associated with high levels of psychological distress and feelings of hostility but also with depression and anger. The one aspect of sleep disruption that seemed to exact the highest toll was trouble falling asleep. It is possible that one of the aspects that make falling asleep difficult is the hormonal shifts that so often occur. We suspect that hormones and menopause in particular can interfere with sleep quality, but the truth is, we don't know exactly why or how. I wish we did—I wish I could tell you that there was a clear link between hormonal changes and sleep deprivation, and that you could just take a pill and solve all your sleep issues. But we're not there yet.

For example, does poor sleep lead to hormone changes, or do hormone changes lead to poor sleep quality? Honestly, we don't know. But we do know that everything works better when we sleep. We know it boosts physical and psychological healing, and we know that hormonal symptoms are less severe with sufficient sleep.

So how do you get this valuable thing called "a good night's sleep"? One of the very best things you can do to help yourself get to sleep later in the day is to exercise earlier in the day. Exercise in the evening is a stimulant and might keep you up, but if *earlier* in the day you've totally exhausted yourself in an exercise class, or running or playing sports or doing whatever you do, then come bedtime, you will be physically exhausted and you are likely to have an easier time falling asleep.

Another problem is the inability to "turn off" your thoughts. This may seem impossible, but what many women don't realize is how much they do to promote an active brain right before bedtime. You want to do just the opposite.

What I tell my patients is that they have to treat themselves the way they would treat a child who is learning how to go to bed at night. If you are having sleep problems, just consider that you've forgotten good sleep habits, and start back at the beginning. We all know those stubborn toddlers who want to keep talking, want another book, want another drink of water, who will do anything to stay up. That toddler doesn't understand what's best for her, but *you* know the importance of a bedtime routine: tubby time, reading a book, shutting off the light, putting on music, getting tucked in, the goodnight kiss. You can do all these things for yourself. The important part of all this is the *ritual*. Ritual is soothing and stress-reducing. Ritual promotes sleep.

This is just one more way to nurture yourself. Think about the things that make you feel calm and relaxed, and create a bedtime ritual around those things. Some ideas that work for a lot of my patients:

- A warm bath. Bubbles?

- A cup of herbal tea (no caffeine!)

- Relaxing music (this is not the time for rocking out to heavy metal)

- A light snack (nothing high-fat or high-sugar), such as an apple with almond butter or a pear with low-fat herbed goat cheese (one of my favorites!)

- A nighttime beauty routine: brushing teeth, flossing, mouth-wash, brushing hair, face cream—whatever you feel you need. Do it the same way and in the same order every time.

- Meditation: When you get in the habit of stilling your mind, you'll be better able to quiet your thoughts so you can sleep.

- Candles with soothing scents like lavender: This can be part of making your bedroom feel like a relaxing spa.

- Declutter your bedroom. Put the work pile in another room, and the laundry that you didn't fold yet out of your sight.

- Sex? Although one study suggested that men sleep better after sex, while women tend to wake up, sex can be a nice way to wind down for many women. If sex does get you wound up, maybe you just need a cuddle or that goodnight kiss.

- Speaking of sex, the bed should be for sleeping and sex only. Anything else can interfere with the process of winding down for sleep.

- Finally, keep electronics out of the bedroom. No TV, no computer. These are also stimulants. If a good book helps you wind down, reading can be part of your routine, but this is not the time to read that page-turning, can't-put-it-down crime thriller.

This is about taking care of *you,* and finding a routine that calms *you* down. The routine itself is the key to relearning how to sleep. You are worth this. Put the kids to bed, then put yourself to bed with just as much nurturing.

Alternative Medicine

You're de-stressing, having sex, sleeping more—great! But what do you do when you aren't feeling well? How do you implement self-care for a cold virus, allergies, arthritis, or something worse?

A lot of my patients ask about alternative medicine, because in their quest to care for themselves, they are curious about what cures they see as more "natural" can do for them. Some of them don't want to be on so many drugs, or they think alternative medicine can act as a preventive, or they just like the idea of having more control over their own health.

I'm not opposed to alternative medicine. As a doctor of osteopathy, I learned to look at a patient as a whole person rather than look at symptoms in isolation, and this is one of the primary tenets behind alternative medicine. I am a proponent of a lot of types of alternative treatments, but I also believe there is an important place for conventional medicine, and in many cases for pharmacologic therapy. I also know that there is quite a bit we don't yet know about alternative medicine, so it is important to use it with caution.

If you're going to use some alternative treatment (acupuncture, Reiki, herbal medicine) instead of conventional treatment, my advice is to do this at the beginning of a disease process rather than when a disease is advanced. Sometimes alternative medicine works very well, even though *we don't know why.* However, it tends to work much more slowly than conventional medicine, so you don't want to use it when the clock is ticking or the disease is advanced. But sometimes you have the time. Your condition isn't that serious yet or isn't necessarily progressive. In this case, alternative medicine might work very well for you.

I had a patient who had hyperthyroidism (an overactive thyroid gland). She had been told it could affect her heart, and she was having a very rapid heart rhythm and palpitations. If you have a very fast heartbeat for too long, it can weaken your heart, so this concerned me. An endocrinologist had told her that she needed to get her thyroid taken out, and she came to me for a second opinion because she didn't want to do something this radical. Instead, she wanted to go to a Reiki practitioner and an acupuncturist and take herbal medicine from a traditional herbalist.

I told her that I would support her doing this (because I could tell she was going to do it anyway, with or without my involvement), but that I would only stay involved under certain conditions. First, she had to put a timeframe on this alternative treatment. We would see each other once a month, and in six months, if she wasn't getting worse, we would reevaluate. Second, if she was getting worse, she would agree to a more conventional approach and consider the thyroid surgery. She agreed.

Six months later, she was not getting worse. She convinced me to let her keep trying her treatment, and because I saw no further decline, I agreed to two more months. Eight months after our first visit, when she walked into my office, I took one look at her and I could tell what was going on. "You're getting better," I said. And she was.

This is what I suggest you do. With guidance from an open-minded doctor, put a time limit on your alternative medicine treatment, and be open to switching to a more aggressive treatment if you aren't getting the results both you and your doctor agree are necessary for your health.

Alternative medicine is not necessarily an either/or scenario.

That's why so many people use more comprehensive terms to describe their treatment plan, like complementary or integrative medicine rather than alternative medicine. You can still use acupuncture, Reiki, homeopathy, even herbal medicine, as long as your doctor knows about it and it doesn't interfere with your conventional therapy (for example, some herbal medicines don't mix with certain drugs).

Let's say you have high cholesterol but no sign of plaque in your arteries, and you haven't had any heart problems. If it interests you and you are motivated to do it, by all means, check out alternative ways of managing your health. See if it works for you. In fact, applying "cures" like diet and exercise is very in line with alternative medicine. A holistic doctor might also suggest certain herbal or homeopathic remedies, or acupuncture, massage, stress reduction techniques, or energy manipulation techniques. Do what makes sense to you. If your cholesterol comes down, good for you! You did it! But if, despite all your alternative interventions, your cholesterol remains very high, then you need to consider doing something more, like taking cholesterol medication. Medication and holistic practices can and should always be used in conjunction with each other. It isn't an "either/or" kind of situation. Using both might decrease the need for higher doses of medication, and at some point may help the effectiveness of the traditional medicine. Just be sure your doctor knows what you are doing.

Alternative medicine can empower you to take your health into your own hands, but part of that power is to recognize when you need more help. Mainstream medicine doesn't have all the answers. I have had patients get better after using acupuncture, Reiki, or transcendental meditation. We can't prove that the alternative treatment did the curing, but I don't believe we can't discount it either.

The fact is that our health-care system is not exactly set up for prevention, and alternative medicine is. We are a reactive medical community. We treat diseases—that's what we've been trained to do.

That's where all the research has been. But things are changing. Insurance companies are restricting payment on testing and medications, medical care is extremely expensive, and people are becoming more empowered to embrace their own health care.

It's up to you to say, "I choose to treat myself this way," as long as you are considering medical opinions in your decision. But get more than one—get two, three, four medical opinions, including holistic medical opinions. Then do what resonates with you. Seek out reputable sources (check out the back of the book for some of my favorites) to help you make an educated and reasonable decision.

Considering all this, I also believe it is very important for you to accept three things when considering alternative health care:

1. Find a doctor who is willing to work with you.

2. Understand that alternative care might help you, but it also might not help you.

3. Have a structured plan, including exactly what you are going to try, how long you are going to try it, and when you will make a decision about whether it is working or not. If it's not working, I hope you will be willing to follow a more conventional approach, especially if your health is at risk.

Supplement Savvy

I know so many women who take supplements for all kinds of things—sometimes they don't even remember what they are for. Some supplements might help you, but others could harm you, so I want you to understand how supplements can be part of self-care, and also how they might not be worth the price tag on that plastic bottle.

I typically don't recommend a lot of supplements because I haven't seen the hard science to support adding them to a healthy diet. Some can react with medications, and some can even make people sick. Supplements aren't well-regulated, and if a doctor doesn't suggest them, you may not have all the information you need to add them to your health-care plan. (And if you do, always tell your doctor and your pharmacist, so everybody knows everything you are taking.)

However, there are a few that probably are worth adding to your diet.

- **Fiber:** Most people don't get enough fiber. A simple fiber supplement can keep you regular (the work of nonsoluble fiber). Soluble fiber has been proven to reduce cholesterol levels.

- **Magnesium:** Magnesium has been shown to help with palpitations and other heart rhythm abnormalities. Most magnesium supplements in stores are made with magnesium oxide. They are inexpensive but not well absorbed. In my experience, the best form is magnesium glycinate. You may need to visit a health food store to find it, or look for it online. A dose of 400 milligrams of magnesium glycinate can help with palpitations, but don't take more than this. Too much magnesium can cause diarrhea. Your magnesium level can be checked by a simple blood test, but the test results don't always reflect whether or not you will benefit from a supplement. Sometimes those annoying extra early beats on the bottom part of the heart (the ventricle) can be blunted with the addition of a magnesium supplement, even if the test doesn't say you are deficient.

- **Omega-3 fatty acid supplements, like fish oil and flax oil capsules:** These are among the few supplements approved by the FDA. Omega-3 fatty acid supplements have a whole host of benefits, from improving the cholesterol panel, lowering triglycerides, and preventing atrial fibrillation, to stabilizing plaque and decreasing inflammation. They might even boost your mood. The recommendation is to take 850 to 1,000 milligrams per day of EPA and DHA (the EPA is the really helpful part, so the more EPA, the better) and for people with high triglycerides, up to 4 grams is recommended.

- **Vitamin D:** Vitamin D could be very important as a supplement if your levels are low. Low levels of vitamin D have been associated with an increase in cardiovascular mortality, high blood pressure, stroke, diabetes, and heart attacks. African Americans are particularly susceptible to low vitamin D levels as a result of decreased sun absorption because of higher dermal melanin. Decreased sun exposure or lower vitamin D intake may account for some of the racial disparities in incidence of heart disease. Have your vitamin D level checked by your doctor at your next appointment. Low vitamin D is a chronic problem, especially for people who live in the northern half of the country. I recommend Vitamin D_3, which is the most bioabsorbable. After taking it for a while, have your levels rechecked. If your levels are low, you often will have to stay on a supplement, but checking the levels is important. Not everyone needs to supplement, and we certainly want to make sure that we don't take too much. Regular recommendations are 400 IU to 2,000 IU daily, or even more for very low levels.

- **B-complex vitamins:** Vitamin B_6 and B_{12} are associated with heart health and keeping the arteries healthy. Sometimes with age, there is a natural decline in the absorption of these vitamins. People who do not eat meat tend to have a low level of B_{12}, because B_{12} is only found in animal products. If you are a vegetarian or vegan, then you might benefit from taking a B_{12} supplement (400 to 1,000 micrograms). Your doctor can check your B_{12} levels with a blood test. Vitamin B_6, found in fish and meat and also in some whole grains, is more controversial in terms of its benefits but potentially helpful. The recommended daily dose is 5 to 50 milligrams, depending on how much vitamin B_6 you are getting in your food.

- **Folic acid**: When taking folic acid, it is also necessary to take a vitamin B_{12} supplement. They work synergistically, and if folic acid is repleted without repleting vitamin B_{12}, it could lead to problems with the nerves. Women who are pregnant should take a folic acid supplement, about 400 to 800 micrograms per day. Folic acid supplementation may be important for heart health, especially if you are not getting it through your diet. However, if you already have a stent, forget this vitamin. It has been shown to increase the risk of blocking up a stent already placed to open a blockage.

- **Coenzyme Q_{10}**: This is an antioxidant that is part of the engine of the cell and part of the energy pathway that generates power and energy in the body. It has been found to be depleted in people taking statins, so I often recommend it if there are side effects of muscle aches or fatigue. It has known to be supportive and helpful for those patients. Studies have shown that it could be beneficial for heart failure, but for those healthy people with good hearts, it is probably not necessary to take. Recommended dose is typically 60 to 300 milligrams per day.

In addition to the few supplements I recommend above, there are some I particularly do not recommend. Here are two to avoid:

- **Do not take antioxidant supplements**: The jury is still out on antioxidant supplements, so I cannot recommend them. The Women's Health Initiative and the Women's Antioxidant Cardiovascular Study (WACS) found no effect of taking vitamin C, vitamin E, or beta-carotene supplements on the risk of cardiovascular events, including stroke or death. It is important to know that buildup of plaque and atherosclerosis probably occurs due to oxidative mechanisms, and in the past we were certain that antioxidants might help to combat this. However, it is impossible to figure out whether taking a supplement for five years can counter the effects of many years of oxidation. It seems that the problem begins at birth, and a measly vitamin just might not be enough to counteract it. Nonetheless, we cannot recommend antioxidant supplements for cardiovascular disease risk reduction because the evidence just isn't there. Yet.

- **Do not take calcium:** Again, the jury is still out on this one, but calcium is not good for heart health and does not protect against osteoporosis or cancer as far as we can tell. The United States Task Force just stated that there seems to be no benefit in taking calcium with vitamin D (these are combined to enhance calcium absorption), even for postmenopausal fracture prevention. In fact, calcium supplements can saturate the receptors in the arteries, and calcium can build up in the arteries, leading to plaque. Stay away from this one, unless your risk of osteoporosis is greater than your risk of heart disease, especially if you are over 65 years old. Talk to your doctor.

Finding Purpose

Finally, I want to talk about something I believe is just as important as sleep or sex or stress. Having it will make all the parts of your life better. It will feed your heart and soul and make you happy. I'm talking about finding a purpose in your life.

I remember early in my career speaking to a large group of people about heart health and saying something to them about how they might feel, and then saying, "Do you know what I mean?" I saw 150 people all nod their heads at me. It was the most incredible feeling, and I remember thinking: *This is it. This is my mission. I want to feel like this every day.*

Ever since then, my passion has been to communicate my message, through television, through writing, through speaking. Along with being a cardiologist, what keeps me motivated on a daily basis is my constant desire to be able to shout from the rooftops: *You can heal your own heart!* and to have the opportunities to really do it. This is the passion that fuels my days, keeps my heart full, and my stress at bay.

Maybe your purpose will be what you do for a career, or maybe it will be something else. It doesn't matter if you make money at it or do it full-time. All that matters is that you have it. Everyone should be able to wake up knowing they have an opportunity to do what they love, and to do what makes a difference, even if it isn't your actual job. This is one of the most important things you can do for yourself. When you find your passion, it's like finding the missing piece in a puzzle.

Think about what gets you excited. What do you love to do more than anything? What is the thing you can think about for hours, that you dream about doing, that you love to tell people about? Follow those clues. It doesn't matter what it is, it just matters that it feels right.

We all have to do things we don't always like. Sometimes you have to take that less-than-perfect job. You have to support your family. You have to make some concessions. But that doesn't mean you can't also do what you love. Make time for it because it matters to you and you are that important. Soon you'll see how much more in control of your own destiny you feel.

I've always believed there are four things that sustain people:

1. Family
2. Love with a partner
3. Health
4. Work with a purpose

If you have all four of those things, then you will have a fulfilling life and a full heart. Nurture your family, whether they are literally related to you or not. Keep your heart open for the one partner who can travel through life with you if you haven't found that person yet. Preserve and protect your health by preserving and protecting your heart. And find your purpose. Whether it's starting your own business or arranging flowers, practicing law or painting, find it! Then share it with others. This will bring your passion full circle. Spread it beyond yourself.

Now that we've talked about self-care and everything it entails, I want to help set you on the right track. I would like you to sit down with yourself and make some lists. You can put these in your Heart Book, or you can write them right here in this book. This is a little exercise to help you begin to turn off your negative habits and start practicing all the things I've been talking about in this chapter so far—optimism, joy, self-love.

First, make a list of ten things you are really happy about in your life. Write them here. Take as much time as you need until you come up with ten:

1. _____

2. _____

3. _____

4. _____

5. _____

6. _____

7. _____

8. _____

9. _____

10. _____

Now, make a list of ten things you are really happy about in yourself. Forget about the things you don't like for now. Just focus on what you believe to be your best qualities. Take all the time you need. If you get stuck, ask a friend about your best qualities. Your friend may see things in you that you aren't seeing.

1. _____

2. _____

3. _____

4. _____

5. _____

6. _____

7. _____

8. _____

9. _____

10. _____

Now, make a list of ten things you are really happy about in your job or choice of employment (this can include the job of stay-at-home mom). Even if you don't like a lot of things about your work life, push yourself to find the things you do like.

1. _____

2. _____

3. _____

4. _____

5. _____

6. _____

7. _____

8. _____

9. _____

10. _____

Finally, make a list of the ten things you would like to change in your life.

1. _____

2. _____

3. _____

4. _____

5. _____

6. _____

7. _____

8. _____

9. _____

10. _____

Think about what you just did. You now have a plan to move forward in your life, led by your heart, not your head. You're getting closer in touch with *you*, including what you love and what you want to change. Now you have the tools to nurture the positives and take action on the changes. Flip the switch. Turn off the dark parts. Find the light in your lists. Find the joyful parts, the gratitude, and the love. No matter what your story used to be, in this new story, you are the hero, and your life keeps transforming and becoming what you most desire.

When you manage your stress, prioritize your sex life, get enough sleep, and consider *all* your treatment options including preventive care, along with the diet and exercise approach I've already recommended, you can feel good about treating yourself well, caring for yourself, and taking your health into your own hands.

This Chapter, by Heart

♥ Stress is often caused by a feeling that you are not in control of your own life.

♥ Optimism is good for your heart.

♥ If you have a passionate purpose in life, you will suffer less from stress.

♥ Get stress under control by mastering the art of well-being.

♥ A healthy sex life is important for quality of life.

♥ Female sexual dysfunction is important to address; it may be a matter of hormone balancing or simply committing to having sex more often.

♥ Lack of sleep is a heart disease risk. Get enough sleep to feel better and be healthier.

♥ Alternative medicine can play an important role in your health care, especially as a preventive or in managing mild problems, but if your health problems are severe, conventional medicine may be preferable.

♥ The ideal approach is to combine alternative and conventional medicine under the supervision of a doctor who is open to this approach.

♥ Try to find your passion and live from the heart, and everything else will fall into place.

CHAPTER THIRTEEN

Hormone Hell

It happens every single month. You make a decision with a little bit more emotion and passion than usual. You get feverishly deliberate about everything you say. Maybe you snap at someone or get the sudden desire to tell your boss exactly what you think of him. Maybe you make a rash purchase or an uncharacteristic decision, or you pour out your heart to someone, absolutely certain you mean every single word with every ounce of your being.

Then you wake up the next morning, and you get your period. You look back over the past week, and you think, "Oh . . ."

And then you wonder how you could have been so wackadoodle nuts. And why on earth, after all these years, you still didn't remember that you get PMS.

If you do get PMS, you may also notice that it's getting worse than it was in your teens and twenties. After age thirty, PMS changes. This is PMS: The Advanced Version, the PMS that hearkens menopause, even if that event is a decade or two in your future. It includes bigger mood swings, more hostility, worse cramping. It makes you a little too harsh, a little too emotional, and takes crankiness to a whole new level. It makes you cry at a sappy TV commercial because that little boy looks just like how *your* little boy used to look (even if he didn't look like that at all), or because that young woman is so thin and pretty, and you used to be thin and pretty and now you're old and you'll never look like that again, or because people try so hard to do the right thing and it breaks your heart, or because your husband doesn't act like that guy bringing his wife her coffee in bed.

You don't sleep well, you don't even want to think about sex, you can't keep your temper under control, and you feel like you don't even know your own mind because your personality seems to change from week to week. Believe me, I've heard it all, I've seen it all—I've *felt* it all. I know.

Maybe nobody ever told you this was going to happen to you. I know that nobody ever explained it to me. But now I know that this crazy time in your life is not your fault. It's the fault of your hormones. Menopause is coming. Welcome to Hormone Hell.

How Hormones Define You

In many ways, your hormones really do define you. From puberty to PMS, pregnancy to perimenopause and beyond, hormones can make you feel good, bad, irritated, depressed, angry, anxious, and yes (let's just admit it), totally crazy! Perimenopausal hormonal shifts start happening in your thirties and forties, and they can do other things to your body besides mess with your emotions. They cause the infamous hot flashes, they can bring on migraines you never had before, and they can mess with your heart. Many women begin to experience heart symptoms for the first time as their hormones begin to shift, and a lot of my patients fear they are going to have a sudden heart attack. Some even fear they are losing their sanity, or at least losing control of themselves, and in many cases I'm surprised to learn that they have no idea hormones are to blame.

Obviously, this isn't a book about hormones, and hormones aren't my specialty, but I see the fallout of Hormone Hell so often in my office that I feel obligated to talk about it. And I hope you won't be disappointed, but the very first thing I'm going to tell you about your hormones is that even though they impact your life dramatically and frequently, the fact is that we still don't understand exactly how they affect our hearts as we age, although the research is being done. We just have to wait . . . impatiently.

We know a few things, and we keep learning more, and the research is addressing many of the unanswered questions about hormones. Back in the introduction to this book, I gave you a list of ten questions from WomenHeart: The National Coalition for Women with Heart Disease and the Society for Women's Health Research that still need to be answered. One of them is about the effect of hormones on the heart. We know there is one, particularly with estrogen, but we don't fully understand the implications of this interaction on the heart. Not yet.

There are hypotheses about how this whole hormonal dance messes with you and causes physical symptoms such as breast tenderness and headaches (usually estrogen related), and how it affects your arteries, the endothelium, and your risk for heart disease. We know that the estrogen of our younger years protects our hearts, in large part because it maintains a high level of that HDL, the good cholesterol. We also know that as we go through menopause and estrogen decreases, so does HDL. Meanwhile, your LDL (the bad stuff) can start to go up, and your cholesterol can increase twofold, rising by 10 to 20 mg/dl. Depending on your lifestyle, you may also be more likely to develop belly fat and elevated triglycerides.

These biological processes continue so that by ten years after menopause, when all of the estrogen is gone from your system, you have about the same heart disease rate as a man.

Another thing that happens due to all these hormonally influenced changes is that those supple arteries that had been so nicely maintained by estrogen begin to get stiffer and less pliable. When this happens, blood pressure increases and arteries become less forgiving in their ability to weather the storm of your lifestyle choices. So now when there are any insults to the endothelium, whether from high blood pressure, high cholesterol, stress, or a lack of exercise, there is more likely to be damage to these stiffened arteries. This ultimately leads to plaque formation. Add to that the fact that postmenopausal women tend to have increased inflammation, which makes plaque more likely to rupture, causing a heart attack or stroke. This is exactly why you need to train for menopause like you are training for a marathon.

In a study of women aged 45 to 60 years, these were the most common hormonally charged symptoms they reported:

- 69% said that hormonal changes were negatively affecting their lives.

- 44% had hot flashes.

- 44% had interrupted sleep.

- 35% had mood swings.

- 34% had lack of sexual desire.

- 27% had vaginal dryness.

- 19% had irregular periods.

Obviously, women are suffering from the effects of hormones, and yet many doctors treat menopausal symptoms either like an illness or as something psychosomatic. Menopause is part of life. It's part of our biology, and I believe it's important to see this as a natural process that doesn't have to be so terrible. If you live a lifestyle more in tune with your body's needs, then menopause will feel more natural too.

But you need to train for it. Let's begin by looking at the stages of Hormone Hell you may be going through right now.

Heart Sense

Fluctuating hormones can wreak havoc on your heart's electric system. One of the first clues some women have that their hormones are fluctuating is heart symptoms. PVCs (premature ventricular contractions) or PACs (premature atrial contractions) often occur with hormonal changes, causing many women to complain of palpitations. The problem is that the only real "cure" is the resolution of hormonal fluctuations. These extra beats won't kill you, but they can certainly affect your quality of life, even waking you up from sleep. I recommend staying hydrated by drinking enough water, staying away from caffeine or stimulants, stopping or greatly reducing alcohol intake, and exercising. Sometimes a magnesium supplement can help suppress these early beats. If they are really bothersome, your doctor can also prescribe a medication to help with the problem.

PMS

Long before you enter perimenopause, you might suffer from PMS, or premenstrual syndrome. This is the period one week before your period, and for many women it's not a nice time of the month. Bloating, breast tenderness, headaches, irritability, and mood swings plague many of us during this time. Nobody is entirely sure why some women have PMS and others don't, but the fact is that many women do.

These symptoms can surprise you every month unless you start tracking your cycle so you always know where you are. Even women on birth control pills might get these symptoms. Although birth control pills can improve PMS symptoms for many women, for some symptoms actually get worse. Of course, it will be naturally easier for you to track your menstrual cycle, since it is artificially regulated by hormones, so at least you'll know when PMS is coming.

For many women, the day they begin to feel crazy is almost always five to seven days before they are due to menstruate. When you know it's coming, you can be prepared. You can remind yourself: *I'm a little crazy right now, so I'm just going to take it easy and hold my tongue and not do anything rash.* It seems ridiculous that we should have to think this, but if PMS happens to you, you probably know who you are and you know this is good advice.

Along with this little mental caution you should learn to give yourself, there are some good ways to ease PMS symptoms. When PMS, or its more severe counterpart, PMDD (premenstrual dysphoric disorder), disrupt your life, your doctor might prescribe low-dose-estrogen birth control. This helps many women by keeping estrogen levels steadier. For others, however, it doesn't help at all, and may even make symptoms worse. You won't know whether this will work for you until you try it.

Lifestyle choices can definitely exacerbate or ease PMS symptoms. The most important and effective ones to try during your PMS week are:

- Avoiding alcohol

- Avoiding caffeine

- Eating plenty of fruits, vegetables, and high-fiber foods

- Sleeping more—sleep deprivation makes PMS symptoms worse!

- Exercise (you're shocked, right?)

The things that are good for your heart are also good for easing PMS, but you might also want to enact a few rules for yourself if you tend to get a lot of emotional symptoms with PMS, and there is nothing wrong with knowing you need to do this for yourself.

For one thing, it's a good idea to keep reminding yourself that when things are bothering you, they will bother you 9 million times more than is realistic when you have PMS. If you *know* this, it can at least help you ride out the storm because when your period starts, you are going to feel more like yourself again. Just keep telling yourself: *In three more days, I'll see this differently. In two more days, I'll see this differently.*

If this is you, then I suggest you also avoid making major decisions during premenstrual week. Avoid volatile conversations if you can. Avoid PMS dialing (the hormonal version of "drunk dialing")! Don't make that call, even though you are just so sure, absolutely sure, that *this is the time to hash out an issue!* It is *not* the time to hash out any issue—not with your parents, not with your estranged friends, definitely not with your ex-husband or old boyfriend. Step away from the phone.

Instead, this is a time to be gentle with yourself, to practice stress management, to go for a walk in the fresh air, to breathe deeply, to try to relax. This is a time to be quiet and introspective, to be extra-vigilant about your healthy lifestyle habits, and to remind your heart that while it may feel extra-open, it may also be a little bit unprepared for conflict.

In fact, this is the *one time* I give you permission to let your head step in and call the shots, because your heart is vulnerable. This is not a time to change your life. You can change your life *next week.*

Your Heart

PCOS, or polycystic ovarian syndrome, is a condition associated with hormonal imbalance that can cause irregular periods, ovarian cysts, and infertility. Polycystic ovaries are covered with cysts, and this condition is associated with a faulty secretion of the sex hormones. People with PCOS often have difficulty metabolizing sugars, so they experience increased levels of insulin, causing the ovaries to generate more androgen, a male hormone secreted by the ovaries. This can cause facial hair growth, hair loss, acne, and increased testosterone levels. Many women with PCOS have metabolic syndrome or diabetes and are obese, because many of the traits of insulin resistance are found in both diseases. PCOS is also associated with elevated triglycerides, and it increases the risk of heart disease. There is some evidence that PCOS can be genetically inherited, but there is also a form that may be related to lifestyle choices.

The exact cause of PCOS is unknown, but about 10 percent of infertile women have it, and it's one of the most underdiagnosed causes of infertility. If you are having trouble getting pregnant, consider checking in with an endocrinologist. Your infertility issues might be related to carbohydrate/triglyceride/insulin resistance issues, and this might be even more significant than any problem with your reproductive organs. The treatment plan is similar to what is prescribed for people who have metabolic syndrome or the ApoE2 gene, because both conditions may involve difficulty metabolizing carbohydrates. Reducing carbohydrates and sugar in your diet and increasing exercise may improve insulin secretion issues, reducing testosterone production and even helping the body to begin ovulating again. This can restore fertility and hormonal balance.

Perimenopause

Perimenopause is the name for the years leading up to menopause. Between the ages 40 and 60, there is a shift in the hormones. During this time, from what we understand, your ovaries, which are usually pumping out estrogen in the beginning of your cycle, are getting tired. This fatigue results in a drop in estrogen production. When you produce less estrogen, your body notices and starts to show some symptoms, including hot flashes, difficulty sleeping, and irritability. When you develop these symptoms, you may be tempted to get your hormone levels checked. However, until your menstrual cycle becomes irregular, hormone tests probably won't show anything. This doesn't mean you are not experiencing perimenopausal symptoms.

As Dr. Susan Love explains it in her book about hormones, back in the brain, where the pituitary gland sits, there are signals that the estrogen is low, and so the brain triggers the pituitary gland to pump out FSH (follicle stimulating hormone), which is the hormone that makes ovulation happen. This spikes up the estrogen release in the ovaries to compensate.

It's like how you can get that burst of frenetic energy when you are at your most exhausted but you know you *must* get something accomplished. That's what your ovaries are doing. This extra estrogen release, which leads to ovulation, also leads to symptoms of excess estrogen, like breast tenderness and headaches, and yes, more irritability. Instead of a nice even flow of estrogen throughout the month, you are getting dips and spikes, and these huge estrogen fluxes are what make you feel so crazy. Also involved is the hormone progesterone, which induces menstruation, and that hormone comes with its own set of symptoms and problems too. But you are not crazy. It happens to all of us eventually. When you do begin to experience menstrual irregularity (skipped periods, or periods at unpredictable times), this is the time to get your hormones checked.

One of the most common treatments for perimenopause is oral contraceptives (birth control pills). These regulate your hormones. Even better, all the lifestyle changes that benefit your heart and that lessen PMS will also help to smooth the perimenopausal transition.

Menopause

When you have not menstruated for one year, this is menopause. It really only lasts a couple of days. You wait, you wait . . . no period. It's been a year. It's official! You are done. You would think there would be fireworks or confetti would fall from the sky, but no, all you get is plummeting estrogen. Then you are officially postmenopausal. Most of the fuss regarding menopause is actually about what happens leading up to it and what happens afterward. When people say "menopausal," they usually mean the year or so right before or after that banner day when you haven't menstruated for one year.

In one study, 2,509 women of multiple ethnicities, ages 45 to 84 years old, including white, Chinese, black, and Hispanic, were followed for an average of five years. Those who reported going into menopause at age 46 or younger had an increased risk of stroke or heart disease, two times greater than those women who went into menopause at an older age. Whether menopause was natural or surgical, the risk of heart disease increased at earlier ages of menopausal onset. Doesn't that make you love your estrogen and appreciate your menstrual cycle that much more?

Heart Sense

Periods of hormonal change are often associated with anxiety, and even more often, with depression. If you have experienced depression in the past, menopause can exacerbate the problem or trigger a recurrence. In menopausal women, depression is a more significant Heart Throb than for younger women and should not be dismissed. If you are having symptoms of depression, please discuss this with your doctor. Depression at this time really stresses the heart. Please ask for help on this one if you can't seem to get yourself out of that funk.

Postmenopause

The postmenopausal time is the time after you have officially gone through menopause, as your estrogen levels continue to plummet until you don't have any estrogen left. We traditionally think of postmenopause being associated with many of the symptoms of decreasing estrogen: loss of libido, vaginal dryness, wrinkling of skin, lack of sleep, hot flashes, and a decrease in memory. You are also at greater risk for heart disease once your estrogen is gone.

The symptoms women have after menopause vary. It all depends on you. Common complaints are hot flashes, mood swings, difficulty sleeping, and vaginal dryness. The truth is that only 20 to 45 percent of women complain of vaginal dryness, and oftentimes women who go through menopause naturally don't experience this as severely as those who go through menopause because of surgery (like an oophorectomy, where the ovaries are removed) or medications (like chemotherapy). Regardless, maintaining an active sex life through menopause is one of the best treatments for some of these symptoms, because having more sex actually affects your estrogen levels. This is a case where "use it or lose it" is an accurate descriptor.

Another extremely important treatment for menopausal symptoms is exercise and an active life. Exercise keeps the heart rate lower, the arteries more flexible, and all the systems that internally regulate the body tuned up. When you sweat and increase your heart rate on a regular basis, your arteries stay flexible and pliable. You may also notice a reduction in hot flashes when you are exercising. Exercise increases the action of the parasympathetic nervous system, whose job it is to stabilize some of these symptoms, like hot flashes. Exercise is one of the best treatments for menopause there is.

You may notice that the symptoms of hormonal imbalance and the treatments for it are all pretty similar, no matter what hormonal stage you are going through, and you are correct. So let's talk about that. What do you do about Hormone Hell, whether it's PMS or post-menopause or something in between?

So What Do You Do About Hormone Hell?

A lot of women don't ask their health-care providers about how to manage their hormonal symptoms, and when they do, less than half say they are satisfied with the discussion. Sometimes the information they get from their doctors is confusing and they don't understand it. Sometimes they get conflicting information and they aren't sure which information sources to trust. Or the doctors just don't know the answers to their questions. That's because this whole subject is confusing and the data are constantly changing. Consequently, what we know about hormones is evolving as we learn more and as the next phase of the Women's Health Initiative and other studies is analyzed. Although this can be frustrating, the fact that we continue to study and continue to learn about it is comforting. We just have to wait for the results!

But here are some basics. I'll tell you what I know.

First of all, I know that the connection between hormones and some of the less quantifiable symptoms, like irritability, mood swings, and emotional upheaval, has not been proven or specifically linked. One study found that emotional instability, irritability, and mood swings are only present as a result of sleep issues caused by hormonal imbalance.

Now, I know this isn't true, and maybe you do too. I know plenty of women who get enough sleep but still experience mood swings, and those who don't get enough sleep but are emotionally steady. If you are a woman between the ages of 40 and 65, you probably know your hormones are related to your moods and brain fog, even without a definitive study to prove it. This is just one of those things that we *know* without having the proof (yet).

But some symptoms have been definitively linked with excesses or deficiencies of specific hormones. The two main hormones that start to get out of balance as you head toward menopause, and that also can do weird things to your body and brain the week before your menstrual period, are estrogen and progesterone. Each one can cause different side effects:

Estrogen is most likely to cause:

- Breast pain
- Fluid retention
- Nausea
- Leg cramps
- Aggravation of a headache
- Sleep issues

Progesterone is most likely to cause:

- Fluid retention
- Bloating
- Headache
- Breast tenderness
- Oily skin
- Acne
- Mood swings

Because they cause all the symptoms, these two hormones are the major components of hormone replacement therapy, so understanding your symptoms can help you understand what hormones might need to be balanced if hormone replacement is indicated (see the next section).

If your symptoms aren't severe and you want to try something more natural, you might find help with some herbal remedies. For many women, taking black cohosh supplements can help. Soy foods can also be beneficial because soy contains a phytoestrogen (plant estrogen) that can help stabilize the estrogen fluctuations. Soy foods are not generally recommended if you have breast cancer, or a strong family history of breast cancer, but they can make a big difference for women who tolerate them. Vitex is an herbal medicine that can be helpful for the symptoms of too much progesterone. Dong quai is another herb that can help balance estrogen and progesterone. Red clover tea and wild yam extract might make a difference. You can also find some remedies on your spice rack, like turmeric, ginger, and flax seeds. If you want to go this route, don't do it on your own. Find a practitioner skilled in herbal remedies, and see what might be best for you.

Some more conventional therapies also might help some of your symptoms depending on what they are. Recently I had a patient come in whom I've known for many years. She would always tell me that she had no libido. I asked her why she didn't feel like having sex, and she thought about it for a while. Then she said, "I just feel so anxious all the time!"

This is so common, and a good example of how the sexual response is both hormonal and emotional, as well as a product of many psychosocial factors. Sexual desire is a complex issue involving all these factors, from biochemistry to psychology. To help her with her anxiety, I prescribed an anti-anxiety medication, which can help stabilize mood biochemically, making the psychological aspect easier to manage. Now we are waiting to see if this helps restore her interest. I am so optimistic that I can't wait to hear about her sex life. She promised she would call me!

Antidepressants might really help some of your symptoms too, especially if you've lost interest in many things you used to enjoy and you feel flat and emotionless. Talk to your doctor about this. Sometimes mood issues during menopause can reflect the issues you often had with PMS. If your PMS is particularly harsh and interferes with your life, you might also talk to your doctor about medication. Premenstrual dysphoric disorder, or PMDD, is a severe form of PMS, and many people find relief with medication.

For some people hot flashes are a real problem, and hot flash issues can last for years! Hot flashes are intermittent feelings of heat, flushing, and sweating on the head and upper torso. Sometimes they're associated with head pressure and sometimes they're associated with heart palpitations. Estrogen therapy traditionally has been a good treatment to minimize hot flashes. Hormone replacement therapy can reduce hot flashes by 80 to 90 percent, but for many people thirty minutes on the treadmill every day may be equally effective. You might think exercise would increase your inner heat, but as I explained earlier, exercise tones the autonomic nervous system, which helps your body control your internal temperature more efficiently, thereby helping to control hot flashes. This works well for many women, although it doesn't work for everyone. However, it will stabilize your mood, help you sleep better, and maintain a younger and more vital you.

The more fluctuations there are in estrogen, the greater the possibility for hot flashes and other symptoms, like insomnia and irritability. For women who are menstruating regularly but who are experiencing menopausal symptoms, including hot flashes, I recommend having your FSH and estradiol levels checked. The FSH levels can fluctuate during early perimenopause, but a high level of FSH and a low level of estradiol are very consistent with menopause and at least validates that you are indeed having hormone-related hot flashes.

Hot flashes and other symptoms can often be treated with lifestyle changes, and many of these are the things you should be doing for your healthy heart anyway:

- Regular exercise (see Chapter 10)

- Stress management (see Chapter 11)

- Decreasing or eliminating caffeine intake

- Decreasing or eliminating alcohol

- Decreasing or eliminating spicy foods (these can trigger a hot flash)

- Quitting smoking

But if you are still miserable, then you should definitely talk to your doctor about whether hormones are right for you.

There is some evidence that selective serotonin reuptake inhibitors (SSRIs) like Effexor, Celexa, Zoloft, Paxil, and Prozac can prevent hot flashes. Although you've probably heard of these drugs as antidepressants, which is their primary function, there is good evidence that they do help some women with hot flashes, especially those who are truly suffering and cannot or don't want to take hormones. If your quality of life is suffering, SSRIs are an option. Within one week of starting an SSRI, the hot flashes should get better. It's worth testing it out for a month or two before calling it quits, but if the medication doesn't help, then talk to your doctor about stopping it.

The fact is, however, that in most cases you don't need a prescription for anything. A healthy diet, regular exercise, stress management, and self-care can make all the difference. I actually had a patient come into my office and say, in a whisper, "I feel really, really guilty. I have almost no hot flashes, maybe for a day or two, but they didn't really bother me, and I still have a sex drive." This woman works out five days a week for thirty or sixty minutes a day and eats a healthy diet. She is living proof that lifestyle management really does help manage these symptoms. But please know, if you are doing everything you possibly can and you still aren't going through menopause as smoothly as you had hoped, then there are options out there for you. You just have to ask your doctor.

Hormone Replacement Therapy

Over the last few decades, hormone replacement therapy, or HRT, has been a huge source of confusion and the subject of intense debate. Because the loss of estrogen is so clearly linked to an increased risk of heart disease, this is a big issue for all of us.

In 1990, the National Institutes of Health established the Office of Research on Women's Health, and it wasn't until then that major causes of morbidity and mortality in postmenopausal women were identified as an important gap in health research. Studies funded by this initiative began to tell us things we never knew before. Although hormone replacement therapy had traditionally been the standard of treatment for hot flashes, we've since learned there are also naturally effective ways to treat hot flashes, such as with exercise, yoga, acupuncture, and meditation, though these approaches don't always work for all women.

When the Women's Health Initiative was launched in 1991, one of their studies included more than 161,000 postmenopausal women over a period of fifteen years. This study's three clinical trials looked at the effect of a low-fat diet that included large amounts of fruit, vegetables, and grains on cancer rates—specifically breast and colorectal cancer—and also on heart disease. The second part of the study looked at the effects of calcium and vitamin D supplementation. The third part looked at hormone replacement therapy on the incidence of breast cancer, heart disease, venous thrombosis (clots), and stroke.

But the researchers ended the third of these trials prematurely because of the link between HRT and an increased risk of heart disease, breast cancer, and stroke, without any health benefits. This study shook the foundation of doctors and women in this country. Prior to this, we believed that estrogen was the wonder drug to keep women vital and healthy past menopause, and the key to reducing postmenopausal heart disease. But what we learned was that sometimes you shouldn't mess with nature. Menopause isn't a disease requiring medical intervention. Rather, it's a natural progression of life, and hormone replacement in older women who really aren't supposed to have estrogen might actually be dangerous.

However, the study was flawed, and it started a panic that was truly unfair and unnecessary. Women panicked, and so did their doctors, stopping all HRT on everyone, with all women believing their lives were going to be cut short. The reality of the study was that only 30 percent of the study population went on HRT before the age of 60, so the study was mostly looking at an older population of women who were more at risk for heart disease and cancer in the first place.

If you are like many of my patients—between the ages of 40 and

60—that study doesn't necessarily apply to you (and even if you are over 60, no study *necessarily* applies to you). People got very upset by the study without paying attention to what it actually told us—and really, it raised more questions than it answered. It told us that heart disease increased in women whose risk was already high to begin with, but it didn't answer the true burning question: what role hormone replacement therapy taken right at menopause and soon thereafter might play in easing the transition when symptoms are the worst and hormone fluctuations most greatly affect the quality of life. All that drama and not enough answers!

The second tier of that trial addressed this topic, and it turned out that there still may be a role for hormone supplementation during the early postmenopausal periods in a way that might actually be protective against heart disease and cancer. Now, this was the part of the study worth waiting for! For example, estrogen replacement therapy proved less problematic than estrogen/progestin treatment, and a transdermal patch provided the lowest risk among types of hormone replacement therapy. For some women, estrogen makes them feel a lot better. Depending on your Heart Throbs, or a family history of breast cancer, it may or may not be right for you, but this is an important conversation to have with your doctor.

Heart Sense

Hormone replacement therapy might help quite a bit right before and after menopause, but hormone replacement therapy isn't indicated during perimenopause. This is the time when your doctor is more likely to recommend an oral contraceptive to help balance out the hormones that you still have. (And to think you used to use it just for birth control.)

The subject is still controversial. Some doctors advise HRT, and others don't. Some say that bio-identical hormones, which are identical to the structure of human hormones, are the safest, and they should be taken in a way that most closely mimics the body's normal hormone production. There are many things to consider when thinking about HRT, and unfortunately, yet again, we don't know all the answers, but here's what I think:

I don't think "replacement" is the right word. We don't need to replace our hormones, because we don't lose them. They naturally decrease, winding down as we move beyond our childbearing years. We don't need to replace anything, because menopause is not an illness. It is a sign of continuing life, and of moving to the next stage.

However, some of us might benefit from hormone *supplementation*. Hormone supplementation just before and after menopause, when you might be having symptoms of severe sleep issues, anxiety, irritability, emotional instability, an irregular cycle, waking up in sweats, or experiencing breast tenderness, might really help you. Depending on your symptoms, your doctor may prescribe estrogen, progesterone (the synthetic version is called progestin), or a low dose of testosterone for a low libido, although testosterone is not part of the standard guidelines. One of my patients swears that a little estrogen and a little testosterone helped her feel like herself again and restored her sex drive.

Only you and your doctor can assess your personal Heart Throbs and the severity of your symptoms, as well as whether your particular symptoms might be eased by some form of hormone supplementation. Considering bio-identical hormones that are exactly compounded for your needs can provide hormonal support exactly tailored to you and may prove to be better tolerated than the pharmaceutical standard dosed brands. But if you have a family history of breast cancer and are predisposed, then taking hormones probably is not the right choice for you.

The current thinking remains that hormones are not recommended right now to prevent disease, but that might be changing too, as recent data has shown that women who do take hormone replacement within the first ten years after menopause actually receive benefits, including reduced heart disease. This is the opposite of what we thought after the Women's Health Initiative and closer to what we thought before it. Information is constantly changing, and sometimes old theories become new again. The bottom line is that hormone supplementation is potentially safe during those first ten years after menopause, so if, despite your efforts to eat a healthy diet and exercise, your quality of life is suffering because of hot flashes, irritability, headaches, breast pain, and what I like to call the "wackadoodles," then consider HRT. Your doctor knows you and your history, so make this decision together. You should both be comfortable with your treatment.

It's All About You

Hormones are so powerful, and I wish that we had a formula to help everyone ease through PMS and perimenopause, but I can tell you this: Part of the problem is that we are still plowing through and pushing through our checklists, running around half-exhausted, and we are never exactly sure if our symptoms are due to perimenopause, exhaustion, or something else we don't even have time to think about.

It's time that we have a conversation about this. If you think you have symptoms of perimenopause but you are not exactly sure, ask your doctor about it. He can test you to see if your hormones are moving in that direction.

But whether or not they are, you know that at some point, they *will*. As long as you are not trying to have one last baby before your time is up, it's okay to just try to live through it, but get ready for it so menopause doesn't come as a surprise or make your life more difficult than it has to. Eat well. Exercise. Reduce your stress. Sleep enough. And *enjoy your life*.

It's up to you. This is life, but only you can decide to make your life easier. Menopause ushers you into a new and wonderful stage of your life, and one of the most interesting things it does as it reduces estrogen and oxytocin and all those other hormones that make you want to tend-and-befriend is to lessen your impulse to put yourself last. This conveniently coincides with the time in many women's lives when their children move out and they no longer need to care for them (there are many exceptions, of course). Women have more estrogen and oxytocin during the childbearing years to biologically encourage the maternal instinct. When the kids are gone, those chemicals naturally decline—it's nature's logical response to the fact that your kids have moved on, but the biochemical process happens whether you've actually ever had children or not. The result is that menopause becomes a time of nurturing the self, or exploring the world, or being able to indulge in deep insights. It's an exciting and rewarding personal time for many women, and you should be able to enjoy it!

This is the time of your life that is about *you*. You can be a little more selfish without feeling guilty, because your hormones aren't driving you crazy with impulses that pull you in every direction. They've been exhausted and they're gone, so enjoy this beautiful time. Going through it gracefully can be challenging, but there are millions of other women who have gone through it and millions more who will.

This is why it's so important to practice a lifestyle you know will ease your transition. Your chances of getting through premenopausal symptoms, menopause, and even postmenopause unscathed and whole and not feeling like you're going crazy are as high as they can be. The hormonally charged stages of your life may not exactly feel like heaven, but they definitely don't have to feel like hell.

This Chapter, by Heart

♥ Hormonal changes can cause many uncomfortable symptoms, including disconcerting emotional symptoms.

♥ Premenstrual syndrome (PMS), perimenopause, menopause, and the postmenopausal period are all times in a woman's life when she probably will have to contend with symptoms related to hormonal fluctuations.

♥ A healthy lifestyle can help balance hormones, and natural remedies like some spices, herbs, and soy foods may also help ease symptoms.

♥ Other interventions may also help some women, including oral contraceptives and hormone replacement therapy (HRT) for stabilizing hormone levels and antidepressants or anti-anxiety medications to help stabilize mood.

♥ Postmenopause is a time to focus on you, and that's a wonderful life stage to anticipate.

CHAPTER FOURTEEN

When Bad Things Happen

I've saved this chapter until now because it is difficult, and yet it's an incredibly important one for heart health, so it's time to address it. This isn't about cholesterol or blood pressure or heart anatomy or even about diet and exercise, but this is very intimately and deeply about your *heart*, so it belongs in this book as much as any other chapter.

Sometimes bad things happen.

Not just inconvenient or slightly depressing things, but things that make you feel like your life is over. You get laid off. Your heart gets broken. You lose everything you own in a fire. You get divorced. You get diagnosed with a terrible disease. Someone you love dies. As a woman, you are also vulnerable to some particular kinds of bad things. Miscarriage. Rape. Traumatic pregnancy or childbirth. Domestic violence. Breast cancer. Ovarian cancer. And the many, many trials that come with being a caretaker.

I know some people who have had bad things happen to them— terrible, unspeakable things—and I'm sure you do too. We don't like to think about these things or talk about these things, but they happen, and when they do, it can feel like your whole world is falling apart, and you don't quite see how you're going to make it. It can feel like trauma, and sometimes it is. After a serious tragedy, heartbreak, or emotional shock, some women can suffer from post-traumatic stress disorder. Forget a healthy diet and exercise—how do you think about the healthiest choice for your dinner or going to the gym when you aren't even sure you remember how to *breathe?*

Many women feel things very deeply in their hearts, and so their hearts manifest dysfunction when their emotions get extreme. I had a patient who was caring for her dying mother, running back and forth between her mother's home and her own, and also taking care of a husband and children and working a full-time job. After her mother died, this woman came to my office. She had severe, rapid atrial fibrillation, going so quickly that I couldn't believe she was walking around.

Another patient of mine who was a professor had high blood pressure and high cholesterol but was normally a happy person who exercised regularly and had a good marriage. Then something happened in the university department where she worked. She got a new boss, who came in and started getting abusive in meetings, making accusations and firing people. This normally calm, happy woman was beyond hyperventilating. She was having severe panic attacks, crying constantly, asking if I could please give her Xanax.

I had another patient whose hairdresser moved out of town without telling her. As silly as it might sound, this left her in a state of panic. She could not stop talking about it or settle down long enough to understand that this was not the end of the world. To her, it really was. Her world was shaken to its foundation. I'd never seen her in such a state of emotional upheaval.

The point is that your tragedy, your trauma, your disaster, is yours. It doesn't matter how it might affect someone else, because it happened to you. By the same token, these are the things in our lives we need to own. Refuse to let tragedy compromise you, and you can transcend it.

And yet many of the people I know who have experienced terrible tragedy or personal trauma turned into amazing, inspirational people. I don't know why some people can ride above the worst possible circumstances while others seem unable to do so, but I do know the ones who make it don't feel like victims. They preserve their essential selves, and they use the bad energy to propel them toward something good. I think we can all try to do this, because every one of us has had some kind of tragedy or heartbreak or just a very difficult period in our lives. For some people, it's adolescence. For others, it's being a young mother and grappling with postpartum depression and losing a sense of who you are. For others, for many women, it happens later, when their marriages fall apart or they lose their jobs or their children move away. And of course, a natural disaster can happen anytime. Anyone can be the victim of a crime. Anyone can unexpectedly lose a loved one.

Whatever it is for you, in this chapter I want to talk about what you can do about it—how you overcome your tragedy and triumph over your adversity. It isn't easy. Oh, how I know it. But it's not impossible either.

My Heart Book

This is an important chapter for me because as a cardiologist, I see the dramatic effects of tragedy on my patients, and as a woman, I've had several times in my life when my resolve and strength were tested. When I first started keeping a Heart Book, I took notes about everyone else, and then one day I realized how important it was to take

notes about myself. As difficult as it was, I realized the critical importance of answering that simple question, "Who are you?"

Today I am a New York City cardiologist writing a book. I am a
spokesperson for Go Red For Women, and I am a mother. But it took
a lifetime to get here, and my story's not over. My story goes on and
on, just like yours does. The more you understand your own story and
what role you play in it, the more you can see all the many possibilities for your future, and the better you can heal your own heart.

When things get really bad, when you get to the point of thinking
you simply can't do it anymore, that's when you really do have to figure out what you need, what matters to you, and exactly who you are.
Your Heart Book becomes a prescription for your own life, if you are
willing to really look at it.

When I look at my own Heart Book, I realize there are things
inside it that I could share, and I've chosen to share a few of them
with you in this chapter. So many of us have similar experiences, and
there are some universal issues that test our resilience and resolve
regarding what is most important to us. We learn from each other,
especially when we can share how to overcome the heartache, by
developing true understanding and by helping each other learn how
to live from the heart. More than anything, when I say, *I get it, I know
what it's like*, you can trust me. You will see that I do.

Career Trauma

When I was a young doctor, there were times that the medical hier-
archy was overwhelming for me. The sleep deprivation became tough,
and I was a sensitive person. The aggressive male environment was
challenging, and it made the rigors of medical training seem more
like the military. At one point, I had reached a level of sheer frustra-

tion and really questioned my choice to continue what I was doing. But something in me wouldn't let me quit. I knew that it would not last forever, as long as I could keep my soul intact.

Part of my difficulty was self-induced. You see, my emphasis as a doctor was so different than what was mainstream in the medical profession. I was so passionate about prevention, but at that time, the "sexy" stuff was about stenting and invasive, lifesaving techniques (we used to consider this very macho, although some of the best interventional cardiologists I know are women). I felt like I was coming from a different planet. The "boys' club" inherent in the medical profession was sending me the message that I didn't belong, and it was hard maintaining my footing. I knew what I wanted to do and was determined to do it, but it wasn't easy. One day I gave a lecture about the endothelium, diet and exercise, stress management, and heart-centered living to a group of doctors who couldn't care less. They wanted to hear about stenting. That was the hot topic. They all looked at me with boredom and disinterest. I was talking alternative and complementary treatments. I was talking prevention. To me, this was cutting edge. To them, it was irrelevant.

After that lecture, I felt like I had hit rock bottom. I remember telling my father that night that no one understood or had any interest in what I was trying to say. I recognized that if I was going to do this doctor thing, I was going to have to try extra-hard, write a little bit more, study a little bit harder. I knew that what I had to say, especially about women's hearts, needed to be heard, but I wasn't sure I could do it. I'll never forget what he told me. He said, "That's great! That means you're onto something. Nothing on the cutting edge is ever accepted at first. You're saying something new." I think my dad was the only reason I was able to go to work the next day.

I was deeply frustrated. I wondered if my work life would ever change or get better. I got stuck in my head for a while and started that downward spiral so familiar to many of us. I wasn't exercising, I wasn't eating right, I was existing on caffeine and sugar, and I was dating someone who wasn't good for me. I was not living from my heart at all. Somewhere along the way, the scale tipped from "stressed" to "bad lifestyle choices" to "I hate my life." When you begin making choices that aren't typical for you, that hurt you, then this is a huge red flag that you are in a bad place. I lost sight of the big picture, which was that I *was* onto something—I had found my calling in life.

Eventually, with the help of some friends and a wake-up call to myself, I realized I was going to have to figure this out, deal with the environment, manage the stress, repair the lack of sleep, and regain control of the whole situation. It was my life, after all. I was going to have to break up with the boyfriend, cut out the coffee and jelly-beans, and go back to the gym. I was going to have to rise above what my head was telling me and listen to that small place inside that said to me that I was exactly where I was supposed to be. It was excruciating at times, but it was also empowering. Being unhappy in a job is one of the most damaging forms of stress, because it involves so much of your time and energy and identity. It can swallow you up. I often hear people complain about jobs that they are not passionate about, a lack of a direction or meaningful work, a boss who doesn't appreciate them or coworkers who make life difficult. Maybe you got fired and you don't have a job, and you know how important it is to have one—financially and emotionally.

So know yourself. Is your job right? Are you at a crossroads? Where do you want to go now? Who do you want to be? Let career trauma open new doors for you. Maybe it's time to make a change, or maybe it's time to double down and get through it with a stubborn tenacity to be who you are no matter what anyone else says. Sometimes things aren't easy, but that doesn't necessarily mean they are wrong. Only you know the answer. Write about it in your Heart Book until you find it inside yourself, and never stop nurturing your heart, by making choices that keep you healthy, especially when you have to make decisions. Keeping your heart present in a career trauma is important in helping you know what your next steps need to be, and you can't do that unless you are taking care of it. That's why heart care has to be a priority when bad things happen, no matter what else is going on in your life.

Brokenhearted

I think many women can relate to the trauma that can come from intimate relationships. Breakups, divorces, infidelity, love lost—these things can break our hearts because we are biologically programmed to want relationships. When they fall apart, it hurts us at a very deep level. I know, because I went through a divorce.

Earlier in this book, I told you about Takotsubo's cardiomyopathy, or broken heart syndrome. This is a sudden surge of hormones brought on by extreme stress, leading to a decreased heart function that appears almost like a heart attack. But profound grief can have more subtle heart consequences too. It can steal you from yourself so you no longer feel like you. It can drain your vitality, erase your optimism, and make you give up on yourself. How do you go from wanting to stay in bed in the fetal position to living your life?

When I got married, I was so in love with my husband, but after a series of crises, including an accident with our son (he's okay now, in case you were worried), our marriage began to fall apart. And then I got pregnant. The timing was horrendous. I had to fly to Michigan to do a presentation for a company that I was a spokesperson for, and I vomited the whole way there on the plane. I did two talks, toured a huge supermarket, then got on the plane and vomited all the way home. As if this wasn't bad enough, I then had a complicated miscarriage, and the effects of that lasted for a very long time. The loss of that pregnancy broke my heart, and at the same time, I was going through a painful divorce, and that broke my heart again. I was doubly brokenhearted, but I knew I had to keep going. I had to keep working. I had to keep being a mother to my son. I had to see my patients. I didn't have any time to grieve or recover, physically or emotionally.

It was difficult trying to overcome the loss of that pregnancy, when life was still there and as busy as always. There was no moment to stop and mourn the miscarriage or process my feelings. I carried that with me for a long time, and I think this happens to a lot of women. The ripple effect from that miscarriage affected so many other things in my life, and the divorce made everything darker and seemingly more hopeless as I grieved the miscarriage alone. By not dealing emotionally with this event, and keeping those feeling inside, my heart rebelled, as it so often does, and that's when I had the supraventricular tachycardia I mentioned in the introduction. My heart was reminding me that it needed some attention.

People don't like to talk about these things—miscarriages and failed marriages and all those "dark side" things in life. But there is a certain reality to being a woman, and it's not all fun and games. We have PMS. We bleed every month. We get our hearts crushed. We go through childbirth. Bad things sometimes happen to our children. We lose pregnancies, and sometimes we lose ourselves. Sometimes we get into bad relationships. Some are physically abusive, and some are mentally abusive, and then we isolate ourselves, because we don't want anyone to know. The reality of what happens behind closed doors is very difficult. We all try our best, but sometimes we wonder how we'll really get through it.

When you are brokenhearted and you don't talk about things or confront and process your inner mess, it will just get worse, and then you get sick. But if you talk about it, write about it, confide in someone, and invest the time to pour out your heart in your Heart Book, you'll be taking care of your heart in a very real and important way.

At some point toward the end of the divorce, I remember having a sudden epiphany. I had survived, and I was still me, even though my heart hurt more than it had ever hurt before. I felt a relief and a sense of happiness that I could feel such a thing as great love and such a thing as great pain. Imagine feeling nothing! Imagine going through all this *life* feeling *nothing*!

That was the day when I asked myself the most vital question: "What happened to me?" I realized that if I wanted to be happy, all I had to do was to go reclaim it. Happiness was my choice. I wasn't asking what happened to the relationship or what happened during this or that scenario when the marriage was falling apart. I was asking, "What has happened to me that will change anything about me tomorrow?"

And the answer was: *Nothing*. Maybe I would have puffy red eyes, maybe bloating from all the popcorn I was eating, but other than that, nothing happened. I was still me.

We feel so devastated when we have heartache and devastation, but think about this: Heartache is *good*, because it means your heart is working. It means you know how to feel. You are *alive*. It is a sign that you were living from the heart, and that's a good thing.

Embrace it—let it wash over you and then let it drain away, and this is what can save you. *Feeling*—deep, painful feeling, heartbreak, despair, these are closely related to joy, ecstasy, and delight. Letting them exist inside you is how you live from the heart. When you shut them away, when your head tells you those feelings don't matter, that's when you lose track of who you are. Feelings are signs that you are being true to yourself, that you tried, even if you failed at something. When you live from the heart, then your heart will begin to mend, even when you feel like it is broken beyond repair.

When you go through something like a divorce or a miscarriage, you really have to be able to say, *This is what matters to me, this is who I am*, in order to get through it. Think about what really matters: your health, your family, your self-esteem, your integrity. And when someone or something pushes you against the wall and forces you to get right down to what is truly important in your life, by breaking your heart or firing you or pushing you away or by whatever other means, that's when you really begin to understand yourself.

Not all of us get that moment, and if you do, then maybe, just maybe, you are one of the lucky ones. Not because the bad thing was a good thing. It was a *bad thing*. I know that. But if you've been through those experiences, it can make you better, not just for yourself but for everyone who loves you.

Heart Beats

Bad relationships are worse for women than they are for men. In fact, women in negative relationships increase their cardiovascular risk by 34 percent, according to a twelve-year study. It is worth getting *out* of a bad relationship if it can't be fixed. I believe negative relationships affect women more than men because of our unique habit of experiencing an event over and over in our heads (you know who you are)—the nuances of an argument, the intricacies of a conflict, how it was said, what should have been said, what wasn't said.

If you monitor the stress response in a woman, you can actually measure the effects every time a woman replays a negative event in her head. It impacts her body, not just when the negative event happened, but every time she relives it. What might be a single stressful event for a man can turn into a thousand stressful events for his wife. I call this the art of perseveration. Letting it go can save your heart, and although it's difficult to break this kind of obsessive habit, it is hurting you, so take control and stop. The bad thing—the argument, the breakup, the heartbreak—happened to you once. And that's enough.

Health Trauma

When I was a second-year medical student, I was sitting in a lecture about breast cancer. I was riveted because one of the other students' wives had just been diagnosed with breast cancer in her thirties and had gone home for treatment while her husband stayed in school. She was a friend of mine, and it was shocking to us all.

I was sitting in this lecture listening, and suddenly I had this strange intuition: Something was in my left breast. I couldn't wait to get out of that lecture hall so I could feel if there really was something there. When I arrived home, I did the self-exam I had just learned about and found a mass, exactly where I thought it would be. What I didn't know then was I had another one in the other breast. I knew what that could possibly mean, and in my twenties, I started mentally preparing for what I had just taken notes on in that lecture.

After a needle aspiration and a biopsy, I had to have surgery. The tumors were not malignant, but it was definitely a difficult time. The surgery was invasive and scary. A woman's breasts are so much a part of what makes her a woman that it is traumatic when they are afflicted with something.

Health crises can make your head tell you lots of stories about who you are. They can make you doubt everything about yourself. They can make you feel weak and vulnerable, and they can make you feel like you have no control over what is going to happen to you.

One of my patients truly opened her heart to me when she shared the story of getting married and moving to another country, after which she suffered through an extraordinarily abusive relationship. She survived and escaped by fleeing the country with her children and was in hiding in the United States. Unbeknownst to her, the man she ran from, who had threatened their lives, found her daughters and contacted them. She feared for their psychological and physical well-being.

During this time, though healthy and fit and only in her late forties, she developed a blocked artery. She had two stents put into her heart within six months but continued to suffer a buildup of plaque around the stents, because the stents were not covering the whole area that was diseased. She came into my office, visualizing that her arteries were manufacturing plaque and there was nothing that she could do. She felt that her body was betraying her and she was going to get sicker. Of course, she was not only dealing with heartbreak and personal trauma but also with this extremely delicate and dangerous heart trauma. I examined her and did some tests, and then I explained something to her that changed her entire way of thinking: Her arteries were not "producing plaque." Putting in the stents could have created some arterial injury, and because of damage to the endothelium, the artery was forming a blockage at the place where the plaque already was, and the original stents weren't taking care of the whole problem.

We would watch it, give her the right medications, and make sure it wasn't getting worse. I told her, "You are visualizing this in the wrong way. You're seeing a heart out of control, manufacturing its own plaque. But look." I showed her the image from her echocardiogram. "See this healthy heart? It's doing just fine. Rewrite your story. You have a beautiful heart; just picture it working the way it's supposed to work. You are healthy!"

I could see her entire point of view shifting. She said, "You mean I'm not sick? I don't have to be sick?" Then she smiled.

In that moment, she transformed from a "sick person" to someone who had control over her health, because she understood what was going on. She realized that all she had to do was take care of herself.

That patient recently came back into my office for a follow-up. She told me that telling her to rewrite her story changed her life. Today her beautiful heart is doing fine.

But sometimes the health trauma isn't yours. It is someone else's—someone you love. When you become the caretaker, you experience a whole different side of health trauma. Playing this role is by far one of the most draining and most stressful of stressors. You do what you need to, but always remember to care for yourself first. So many of my patients are caretakers, so I see the effect this stressor has on the heart. Almost without exception, the problem is that they are not taking care of themselves.

Without self-care, you cannot help anyone else. Make your own checklist for the day, before you start running in circles to care for someone else. Put your own oxygen mask on first. It's the only way you're going to make it, and others are depending on you, so *you have to make it*. Do what it takes to save yourself, or you are no good to anyone.

Your Survival Strategy

Standing your ground against the odds, finding your voice in a man's world even though you're a girly girl, having difficult pregnancies or miscarriages, going through a divorce, becoming afflicted with a health issue or becoming a caretaker—these aren't paths most of us would choose. You won't always take the easiest path, even by choice, but your path is yours, and it makes you who you are. If you survive it.

So you have to have a plan. What is your survival strategy? When bad things happen, how are you going to make it to the other side?

There was a moment in time when it occurred to me that everything that happened to me happened so that I would be better able to understand my patients and all the women who came to me for help.

I told myself that by going through these issues, I understood, I could empathize, and I could share my story so other women wouldn't feel so alone. I could show women that they too can survive, and even thrive. Maybe this was a survival mechanism, telling myself I had to go through all of this for the good of others, but it worked for me.

And it was true. Now I do feel like I can genuinely empathize with anything my patients have to endure. Sometimes I feel like I can empathize with any woman who walks into my office, because I've been through so much. I *get* the "woman thing." I know how things like breast surgery and miscarriage and C-sections and emotional humiliation affect your sense of yourself and your own femininity.

I look back and remember overcoming each obstacle, and because of that, I can say that each experience provided new lessons and a deeper understanding about who I was. My life has given me the ability to understand many of the issues that women face. I'm glad I know what it feels like to love passionately and to feel great pain. This is how I survived, and if telling you helps you even a little, then it was worth recording some of my Heart Book in *this* Heart Book.

So when you write in your Heart Book, let it be that place where you find *your* will to survive. What is your mechanism? How will you make it okay for you? Why is this happening to you? Give it a reason. Give yourself a purpose.

Write it: This is happening to me because _____.

This is what I'm going to do with this experience: _____.

Everyone needs to feel some power over their lives, some control. The best way to do that is to turn around and remind yourself that you still have *you*. That's very hard for some people who don't think they are so great, but that's why you have to evaluate yourself in a way that you may never have before. When you hear people say, "Work on yourself," you might wonder what it means, and I'll tell you: It means the person you rely on, the person you have confidence in, has to be *you*, first and foremost. You have to feel safe and nurtured by *you*. You have to love who you are. Do what it takes to believe that.

We tend to think the people who know us best are our loved ones, but then I think of how my patients have occasionally said things while going through a divorce such as, "I was married for thirty-five years and I didn't even know him." Don't get to the end of your life and realize you never really knew your own heart. You are the only one who really, truly knows *you*.

You are the only one who can live from your own heart. You are the only one who knows what your heart feels like. No one else will ever have the words to describe your heart. The answers are within. You just have to bring them out.

How to Change Course

When bad things happen to you, I would like you to try something. Sit back and see if you can determine how much you might be participating in the situation. I don't mean you are to blame. I don't mean you *caused* the bad things. I've had many bad things happen to me that I didn't cause. I miscarried. That wasn't my fault. My son was in an accident. That wasn't my fault. But what was I doing to torture myself about the things going on in my life? How was I participating in perpetuating the bad feelings *about* the tragedies?

This is a perception issue. When bad things happen, it's very easy to slip into the role of victim. "Why me?" can quickly turn to "Woe is me!" And then you start thinking, "What's next? What bad thing is going to happen next?" You start bracing for the next big disaster. You start to expect it. And then they come, one after another.

During this harsh time in my life, a friend sat me down and gently asked, "What's with the victim thing?" Despite my insistence that I didn't feel like a victim, his accusation resonated. And it stopped me in my tracks. Sometimes situations occur when you have to force yourself to ask what you are doing to make things go from bad to worse. Then you have to ask yourself how you can stop doing it. Even though we don't have control over many of the misfortunes in our lives, how we choose to negotiate them, from a place of power or from a place of victimhood, can make a difference in how we perceive the situation in the first place and how well we recover.

I spend a lot of time in this book telling you that you have the power to change your life, and I mean that now as well. You can arrest the progress of negativity in your life. We all go through hard times. Instead of thinking about what terrible thing is going to happen next, start wondering what the next wonderful thing will be. That puts your heart in a totally different place.

I see a lot of my patients going through this: Whether they are plunged into despair by the diagnosis of heart disease or whether other bad things happen in their lives, this is when the chest pain starts. This is when the palpitations start. Your heart is throwing up a red flag. It is your alarm system. Are you listening? No matter what happened, it was part of your journey, so you have to make peace with it in order to move forward. Remember those people who come out of tragedy better for it, no matter how bad it was—people who change the world because they realize how hard life is, and they want to help others get through the darkness? This could be you. Move toward the light in your life. You don't have to keep going deeper in.

When I think about my marriage and my divorce, without regret I can say that the best thing I ever did was marry him, and yet the best thing I ever did was divorce him. Every *heartfelt* thing you've ever done in your life is the best thing you ever did. All the painful situations you've endured or choices you made have to be what they are, without remorse, regret, or shame. It had to happen because it did happen.

This is how you reclaim your power. This is how you stop feeling like a victim. You do the best you can every day. You think about what you want, and you live from the heart. You think: *How can I be the best me I can be every single day, no matter what happened yesterday? How can I nurture my body and my soul?*

When you begin to think like this, then you might not feel so compelled to drown yourself in ice cream or doughnuts or an entire bottle of wine. You might even feel like going for a walk. You might call a friend or a therapist. You might start to see that you can love yourself and act accordingly.

I think it's natural to try to avoid feeling bad. Working women in particular have learned to bury their emotions and move on, but you need to let it out. Deal with it, and only then will it be gone. Let yourself feel the sadness, the anger, the hurt. *It's okay to feel hurt.* Go ahead and wallow. Take twenty-four hours. Take a week. Take what you need, but no more. Go ahead, sob on the bathroom floor. Feel. Your heart is working, so good for you. Now, pick yourself back up and start taking care of yourself. It's time.

You don't have to do it alone. I urge all of you to find your people, build your village, and get help from friends, therapists, or healers.

Learning who you really are and then taking care of yourself the way you deserve justifies everything else in your life. It justifies the lessons you learned. It justifies the effort, the joy, and especially the self-love.

Recently I received a phone call that upset me. There was not much I could do to change the situation or make it better. I could have fretted, tortured myself, lost sleep. But I didn't. Instead, I took a Pilates class, and then I walked home listening to music on my iPhone. Headphones in, I was literally dancing down the street. I can't tell you how happy that made me feel. I was right back to being 17 years old, listening to '80s music. I didn't care who looked at me. I used to be a dancer, and I was dancing! It was *me*! I was wearing this huge hat and sunglasses, and I can't even imagine what people thought of that crazy lady, but at that moment I didn't care. I felt carefree and happy and whole. This is what I want for you. Maybe you won't look as silly as I did, but I want you to find joy again.

I want you to find yourself. Look for her, especially in those moments you most fear she has slipped away. She's in there. She's in your heart. Find that place in you that you loved when you were young, when you were a child, happy and carefree, and let it heal you. Let yourself feel your own love. Be there for yourself.

Put on your headphones and dance down the street.

This Chapter, by Heart

♥ Sometimes bad things happen, and they can hurt your heart.

♥ When you face trauma, tragedy, death, or the end of a relationship, you can feel like it is impossible to go on, but you can devise your own survival strategy.

♥ If you find a reason for what you've endured, you eventually will be able to triumph over your tragedy.

CHAPTER FIFTEEN

Open Your Heart

About a year ago, someone asked me what I like most about myself. I thought for just a second, because the answer was simple: I live from the heart. I don't always make the right decisions, and sometimes I make blatant mistakes, but I live from a place where what I do matches what I think, what I feel, my values, my truths, my weak points and strong points. I live from a place of knowing that my choices will help support me in being the best I can be.

When you stop and ask yourself what you like most about *yourself*, what's your answer? No fair saying that you are a good mother, or a giving wife, or that you love your family, or that you are excellent at your job. Those are all about what you do and your relationships to others, important as those are. What I'm getting at, what I'm really asking, is: What is it about you that makes you who you are? It's the part that has always been with you, the part that was you at the age of 6 and 16 and 26 and all the way until now.

Many years ago, my mother and I were driving back from Missouri to New Jersey for Thanksgiving break. I was in medical school in Missouri, and it was the Thanksgiving holiday. There was a horrendous snowstorm and we couldn't see where we were going. All we knew was that we had to keep driving in order to make it home on time for Thanksgiving. Prior to the trip, I got snow tires and special windshield wipers to wipe off the heavy snow. We packed up the car. We thought we were prepared and ready, but nothing could have prepared us for the Midwestern blizzard. While we were driving on the highway, trucks were zooming by with the snow flying out from under the flaps around their huge tires. There we were, puttering along in the right lane, and every time a big semi passed us, we would get completely blinded by the snow.

My mother drove first, and the first time this happened—this virtual blinding by the racing, slush-hurling semis—we both screamed. We realized that within ten seconds, we had full visibility back, but this only slightly calmed us. The second time it happened, we counted to ten and my mother said, "We did it! Made it again!"

By the tenth time, we drove as if we barely noticed the slap of slush across our windshield, chatting together as if such a thing were perfectly normal—to be hurtling through the dark blizzard on the interstate with zero visibility. Because we weren't going to stop. We had a goal. We wanted to get home.

This is how I see the journey toward health and wholeness. Every single one of us has inside of ourselves this organ, this amazing machine that not only sends blood and oxygen throughout the body, but that is the metronome of our lives. How we live nurtures this vital organ, or hurts it. We don't always know what life will hurtle at us, but if we have a goal, we can keep going, even when we are flying blind.

Maintaining heart health isn't just about preventing heart attacks and strokes. It's not just damage control. It's not stopping the car and wiping off the windshield every time a semi hurtles by. It's going forward, sticking to a lifestyle you know will make you a better person, even when you don't feel like you understand why at any given moment things aren't going the way you planned. It's doing the right thing, even when it's hard, or you are tired, or you want to binge on sugar, or your windshield is covered in slush. This is living from the heart—feeling your life rather than thinking your way through it. Knowing the road is still there under your tires, even when you can't see it. Having faith.

Another situation that I will never forget happened while I was snow skiing. I saw a mother, a father, and a little boy getting on the chairlift. The little boy fell off right at the start. The parents were so engaged in their conversation that they were a bit ahead when they noticed. The lift operators did not see him, because he was on the ground. The little boy stood up exactly where he fell off and got hit hard in the head with the next empty chairlift coming toward him. He fell again, but instead of staying down—and by now, everyone was screaming at him to stay down—he got up again, right under the chairlift in the same place, and got smacked in the head by the next chairlift. By the time the third chairlift came, the operators shut down the equipment and picked up the near-unconscious child. This image has stayed in my mind for almost twenty-five years.

I think about that little boy whenever I have a patient who keeps living in a way that hurts her heart, even when all the information around her is telling her to stop those unhealthy habits that are like that chairlift knocking the little boy down over and over again. Figure out what is good for you, what nurtures your life and your heart, and wrap yourself in that world of health and happiness. When an action, a choice, a lifestyle decision makes you feel smacked in the head, as if you have no control over what's happening to you, this is when you change what you are doing. That little boy on the chairlift was just a child. He didn't understand that he shouldn't keep getting up in the same place. But you are no longer a child, and you can decide to make a change—to protect your head, your heart, and your whole being.

Think about this: If you have gotten yourself into a place of ill health, or just a lack of vitality, how did you get here? How many times did you choose to do something that hit you over and over again, only to hurt you? It could be the way you eat, the way you don't exercise enough, the way you let stress hijack you, the way you choose relationships that don't support you, the way you isolate yourself, the way you feel guilty about having fun. Any of it! Stop doing it.

In exactly the same way, this book is me, screaming to you to stop doing the things that are hurting you. I'm calling out to you based on my experience, my passion, and my desire to help you: Stop doing the same painful thing over and over again! You can help yourself. You can live the life you choose to live. You can.

I have been surrounded by extraordinary people, some of whom have overcome extraordinary situations to become who they are. I have a group of wonderful patients who have shared their hearts with me, their trust, their health, and their lives. I feel honored to have been given the opportunity to know them. Each and every patient has affected me, changed me, and brought me to this place today. But they only changed me because I let them change me.

You are not a passive participant in your life, and you are not a victim. Every situation and everything that happens to you is part of your journey to becoming the best possible *you*. Search your own heart to find and unlock your passions and dreams, and know that all you need is an action plan, a desire, and a true willingness. Always be honest with your own heart. Keep yourself accountable. And thrive.

There is a magnet on my refrigerator that I read often. It is a quotation by the author Asha Tyson. It says:

Your Journey has molded you for your greater good, and it was exactly what it needed to be. Don't think that you've lost time. It took each and every situation you have encountered to bring you to the Now. And now is right on time.

This is exactly how I see my life. What happened needed to happen. I wasn't wasting time. I wasn't making mistakes. I was *living*, changing, and becoming myself, and so are you living, changing, and becoming yourself. But who do you want to become?

Many times throughout the years, when things were tough, when I had to do a procedure on a patient that was challenging, or I personally had to endure situations that were difficult, I thought about my mother and that stormy night so many years ago. I thought about how, over and over, we "made it again!"

In a way, it felt like we were cheating death together, but it wasn't a cheat. We were as prepared as we could be. We took all the steps we needed to take to make sure that we would be safe. We did the best we could to be ready for the situation. We did everything to help ourselves. And then we trusted that it was all going to work out. We did get home that night. We made it all the way.

Living from the heart means really knowing who you are, knowing what makes you happy, knowing your strengths and weaknesses, knowing what makes you tick, and understanding that while you are not perfect, you can be as perfect as possible. This is my wish and challenge for you: Live truthfully, authentically, and honestly, drawing strength and consolation from work, family, love, and health. Cultivate and nurture those things, not from your head, where logic always rules, but from your heart, where you can feel what is right and real for you. Live that way, and chances are things are going to be just fine.

This Chapter, by Heart

♥ Always live from your heart.

♥ Your head will tell you a lot of things, but your heart will always tell you the truth, if you really listen.

♥ Let yourself learn from your own life, especially your "mistakes."

♥ Each experience is part of your story, so never put yourself down, do things that hurt yourself, or lose track of who you are.

♥ Everything that happens to you happens for a reason. Find out the reason, and become the best possible you.

♥ Always pay attention to and nurture your heart. Once you decide to live from the heart, the rest of your life will blossom.

Dr. Steinbaum's Meal Plan

I am not a cook. Period, end of story. I do believe in healthy foods, and am insistent on making sure that my son and I have a healthy, nutritious diet.

So, knowing full well that I am not a cook and that I do not like cooking, believe me when I say that you can eat this way too. You can put together these meals if I can. Trust me. I am not saying these are extravagant or gourmet, but they are what to eat when you don't have time or the inclination to get fancy in the kitchen and you want to be healthy, or you're just too exhausted to figure out anything else. I've given you seven options for the seven days of the week. Mix and match or investigate other sources for a plant-based diet, which is the way I eat.

If you do want to add some lean meat to this diet, that's also fine. I recommend chicken and turkey, as well as fish (which I do eat sometimes). If you eat fish, enjoy it two or three times per week for maximum benefit. I do not think anyone who wants a healthy heart should eat red meat. And don't even ask me about bacon. Bacon is not a food. Pretend you never heard of it.

I hope you enjoy these meals. They certainly work for me.

Breakfast

- Spelt bread with pumpkin butter and apple butter. It's like having an apple pumpkin Thanksgiving for breakfast!

- Multigrain bread, sliced low-fat mozzarella cheese, sliced tomatoes, and basil leaves

- Oatmeal, flax seeds, blueberries, ½ teaspoon agave nectar

- Greek yogurt, blueberries and raspberries, with Wasa bread and almond butter

- Ezekiel multigrain wrap with egg-white omelet with mushrooms, spinach, and goat cheese

- Multigrain bread with beets, goat cheese, and dill

- Vegetable scramble with 1 yolk and 2 whites with scallions, tomatoes, mushrooms, spinach, and sautéed kale (use 1 tablespoon olive oil)

Lunch

- Arugula with grilled salmon

- Mixed greens with chickpeas, red beans, quinoa, and balsamic vinegar and black pepper

- Vegetarian pea soup with multigrain bread or crackers

- Steamed broccoli over whole-wheat couscous, topped with grilled tofu

- Spinach salad with tofu, chickpeas, red beans, beets, carrots, corn, broccoli, and balsamic vinegar and olive oil, seasoned with pepper and a dash of salt

- Multigrain bread with avocado and sardines (in water)

- Avocado, tomatoes, and spinach (optional: add low-fat cheese) on multigrain or spelt bread (optional: mustard)

Dinner

- Steamed kale seasoned with pepper and lemon juice, goat cheese crumbles over whole-wheat couscous

- Sautéed vegetables like green and red peppers, scallions, tomatoes, broccoli, cauliflower, and carrots with 2 tablespoons olive oil, add Mrs. Dash seasoning to taste (non-salt seasoning), and mix with quinoa.

- Crushed tomatoes in a pot with pepper, salt, oregano, and garlic to taste. Pour over quinoa pasta. Steam broccoli, kale, or anything green to eat on the side.

- Grilled salmon over steamed kale or collard greens

- Grilled romaine lettuce brushed with olive oil and sprinkled with garlic and pepper, with grilled tofu

- Eggplant and tomato cubes and zucchini slices baked on a baking sheet with salt, pepper, and olive oil (bake at 350°F for 25 to 30 minutes), then tossed with chopped parsley, lemon zest, and fresh lemon juice. Serve over whole-wheat pasta. (This recipe is from, my manicurist, Aurora.)

- Chickpeas (1 can, rinsed well) blended with 2 tablespoons olive oil, salt and pepper to taste, fresh lemon juice, and minced garlic to taste. Serve with sliced fresh tomatoes, cucumbers, olives, and onions, along with toasted whole-wheat pita bread wedges. (Also from Aurora.)

Snacks

- Low-fat or air-popped popcorn

- Blueberries—I eat them like potato chips

- Raspberries

- Pears with a tiny dab of pepper goat cheese (this snack makes me feel like I'm in Paris)

- Apples with almond butter

- Almonds or pistachio nuts—I always keep these in my office desk for those times when I know I have to go a long time without a meal. I don't keep nuts at home or I will overeat them.

- Whole-grain or multigrain crackers

- Raw vegetables like celery and carrots

- Edamame

- Dark chocolate. I have dark chocolate every single day, always 70% cocoa, I don't care what brand. I usually have half of what is recommended on the package for a serving, which translates to one or two squares.

MA'S SOUP

My grandmother, otherwise known as Ma, supplied my grandfather and the rest of her family with many nutritious meals. This soup is nutritious and delicious, and it freezes well, so make a big batch for a big group of people, or freeze portions for yourself so you can always have a good meal when you need one. This is health in a bowl, and it is the one thing I will actually bother to spend time cooking. It reminds me of my home and childhood.

You can find the mixed-bean vegetable soup mix in the soup section of your grocery store—it comes with a variety of dried beans and a seasoning packet.

Mixed-bean vegetable soup mix

1 large onion, cut into quarters

1 cup diced carrots

1 cup diced celery

1 cup diced parsnips

1 cup diced string beans

½ cup dried lima beans

¼ pound fresh mushrooms, sliced

4 cloves garlic, diced

1 cup barley (hulled or pearl)

Any other legumes or beans that you might like

Salt and pepper to taste

Combine all the ingredients in a large stockpot with four quarts of water. Bring to a boil over high heat. Reduce the heat, cover, and simmer for 2 to 2½ hours, adding more water if needed.

Grocery Shopping by Heart

Sometimes the first step in taking care of your heart is to have the right food at your disposal. Now, clean out the pantry and the refrigerator and get rid of all that unhealthy stuff so you can make room, and get ready for eating to care for your heart.

This grocery guide, courtesy of Go Red For Women of the American Heart Association, will help guide you through the supermarket as you stock your kitchen with the heart-healthiest foods. If you choose to be vegetarian or vegan (which I generally recommend), forgo animal products in favor of high-quality plant proteins like tofu, tempeh, edamame, and more legumes like lentils, black beans, and white beans. Use nut butters in moderation, as they are high in protein but also high in fat. Always have olive oil and canola oil in the house. (Canola oil is better for cooking.)

VEGETABLES

☐ Asparagus ☐ Corn on the cob

☐ Broccoli ☐ Eggplant

☐ Cabbage ☐ Green beans

☐ Carrots ☐ Peppers

- [ ] Potatoes
- [ ] Spinach
- [ ] Squash

FRUITS

- [ ] Apples
- [ ] Apricots
- [ ] Bananas
- [ ] Blueberries
- [ ] Cantaloupe
- [ ] Grapefruit
- [ ] Honeydew melon
- [ ] Nectarines
- [ ] Raspberries
- [ ] Strawberries
- [ ] Watermelon

MEAT/POULTRY/FISH

- [ ] Extra-lean beef/pork
- [ ] Fish
- [ ] Skinless chicken/turkey

BEVERAGES (THE BEST IS WATER, BUT IN THE EVENT YOU WANT SOMETHING ELSE . . .)

- [ ] Low-sodium tomato juice
- [ ] Low-sodium vegetable juice
- [ ] Natural/hand-squeezed orange juice
- [ ] 100% juices—no sugar added

CANNED GOODS

- [ ] Beans and lentils
- [ ] Low-fat/low-sodium soups

- [ ] Low-fat water-packed chicken
- [ ] Low-fat water-packed tuna
- [ ] Low-sodium pasta sauce
- [ ] Low-sodium vegetables

DAIRY

- [ ] Egg substitutes
- [ ] Fat-free nondairy cheeses
- [ ] Low-fat or fat-free yogurt
- [ ] Low-fat or skim milk
- [ ] Low-fat ricotta

SNACKS/DESSERT

- [ ] Almonds
- [ ] Hazelnuts
- [ ] Low-fat, trans-fat-free cookies
- [ ] Macadamia nuts
- [ ] Plain, unsalted popcorn
- [ ] Sorbet or low-fat ice cream
- [ ] Unsalted pretzels

BREAD (PITAS, DINNER ROLLS, ENGLISH MUFFINS, WRAPS)

- [ ] Light breads
- [ ] Multigrain breads
- [ ] 100% whole-wheat bread
- [ ] Small slice breads
- [ ] Whole-grain bread

PASTA/GRAINS

- [ ] Brown rice
- [ ] Quinoa

☐ Whole-wheat blend pasta

☐ Whole-grain pasta

BREAKFAST FOODS

☐ All-Bran cereals

☐ Steel-cut oatmeal

DELI DEPARTMENT (CHOOSE LOW-FAT, LOW-SODIUM)

☐ Lean chicken breast

☐ Lean ham

☐ Lean turkey

More Resources for Heart-Smart Women

BOOKS

Balch, Phyllis A. *Prescription for Nutritional Healing*. Fifth edition. New York: Avery, 2010.

Brand-Miller, Dr. Jennie, and Kaye Foster-Powell. *The Low GI Shopper's Guide to GI Values 2012: The Authoritative Source of Glycemic Index Values for Nearly 1,200 Foods*. Boston: Da Capo Press, 2012.

Campbell, T. Colin, and Thomas M. Campbell. *The China Study: The Most Comprehensive Study of Nutrition Ever Conducted and the Startling Implications for Diet, Weight Loss and Long-Term Health*. Dallas: BenBella Books, 2006.

Cloutier, Marissa, and Eve Adamson. *The Mediterranean Diet*. New York: Harper-Collins, 2004.

Esselstyn, Caldwell B., Jr. *Prevent and Reverse Heart Disease: The Revolutionary, Scientifically Proven, Nutrition-Based Cure*. New York: Avery, 2007.

Fuhrman, Joel. *Eat to Live: The Amazing Nutrient-Rich Program for Fast and Sustained Weight Loss*. Revised edition. New York: Little, Brown, 2012.

Gonzalez-Wallace, Michael. *Super Body, Super Brain: The Workout That Does It All*. New York: HarperCollins, 2012.

Jamieson, Alexandra. *Vegan Cooking for Dummies*. Hoboken, NJ: Wiley Publishing, 2011.

Kaminoff, Leslie, and Amy Matthews. *Yoga Anatomy*. Second edition. Champaign, IL: Human Kinetics Publishers, 2011.

Maizes, Victoria, and Tieraona Low Dog, editors. *Integrative Women's Health*. New York: Oxford University Press, 2010.

Miles, Pamela. *Reiki: A Comprehensive Guide*. New York: Tarcher/Penguin, 2008.

Ornish, Dr. Dean. *Dr. Dean Ornish's Program for Reversing Heart Disease: The Only*

System Scientifically Proven to Reverse Heart Disease Without Drugs or Surgery. New York: Ivy Books, 1995.

Rosenthal, Norman. *Transcendence: Healing and Transformation Through Transcendental Meditation.* New York: Tarcher/Penguin, 2011.

Rubin, Gretchen. *The Happiness Project.* New York: HarperCollins, 2009.

Serure, Pamela. *Take It to Heart: The Real Deal on Women and Heart Disease.* New York: Morgan Road Books, 2006.

Stone, Gene, editor. *Forks over Knives: The Plant-Based Way to Health.* New York: The Experiment, LCC, 2011.

Williamson, Marianne. *A Woman's Worth.* New York: Ballantine, 1993.

DIET-RELATED WEBSITES

American Dietetic Association: www.eatright.org

American Heart Association: www.heart.org

Eating Well magazine: www.eatingwell.com/blogs

Everydiet: www.everydiet.org

Fitday—free diet and weight-loss journal: www.fitday.com

Food Network—recipes and information for heart-healthy foods: www.foodnetwork.com/heart-healthy-foods/package/index.html, blog.foodnetwork.com/healthyeats

Nutritient Rich: www.Nutrientrich.com, www.nutrientrichfoods.org

EXERCISE-RELATED WEBSITES AND APPS

www.ABC-of-Fitness.com

American Council on Exercise: www.acefitness.org

www.ExRx.net

www.Fitness.com

Startwalkingnow.org

App: MyFitnessPal

App: iTreadmill:Pedometer Ultra w/ PocketStep

HEART-RELATED WEBSITES

American Heart Association, Go Red For Women: www.goredforwomen.org, www.heart.org, blog.heart.org

American Osteopathic Association: www.osteopathic.org

Black Women's Health Imperative: www.blackwomenshealth.org

Centers for Disease Control and Prevention: http://www.cdc.gov/healthyliving

Events of the Heart—educating and empowering women through the performing arts, "The Angina Monologues": www.Eventsoftheheart.org

Evidence-Based Guidelines for Cardiovascular Disease Prevention in Women: http://circ.ahajournals.org/cgi/content/full/115/11/1481

Healthfinder: www.healthfinder.gov

Heart Healthy Blog: www.hearthealthyblog.com

National Coalition for Women with Heart Disease: www.womenheart.com

National Heart, Lung and Blood Institute: www.hearttruth.gov

National Institutes of Health, Office of Dietary Supplements: http://ods.od.nih.gov

National Women's Health Information Center: www.womenshealth.gov

North American Menopause Society: www.menopause.org

Office on Women's Health: www.4woman.gov

Self Magazine's Heart Health Blog: www.self.com/health/blogs/nutritiondata-heart -health

Women's Health Initiative: www.nhlbi.nih.gov/whi/

WomenHeart, The National Coalition for Women with Heart Disease: www .womenheart.org

SELF-CARE WEBSITES AND APPS

Reiki, Medicine, and Self-Care: www.reikiinmedicine.org

http://www.mindbodygreen.com

Massage information: www.amtamassage.org

Yoga: www.yoga.com

Yoga Finder: www.yogafinder.com

www.thebreathingproject.org

www.vitalaffirmations.com

App: All-in YOGA HD: 300 Poses & Yoga Classes by Arawella Corporation

App: iYoga+ by Breitschmid Productions

App: Universal Breathing—Pranayama by Saagara

App: Relax & Rest Guided Meditations by Meditation Oasis

Index